WORKBOOK

Medicine
—— for the ——
MIND
Common Core

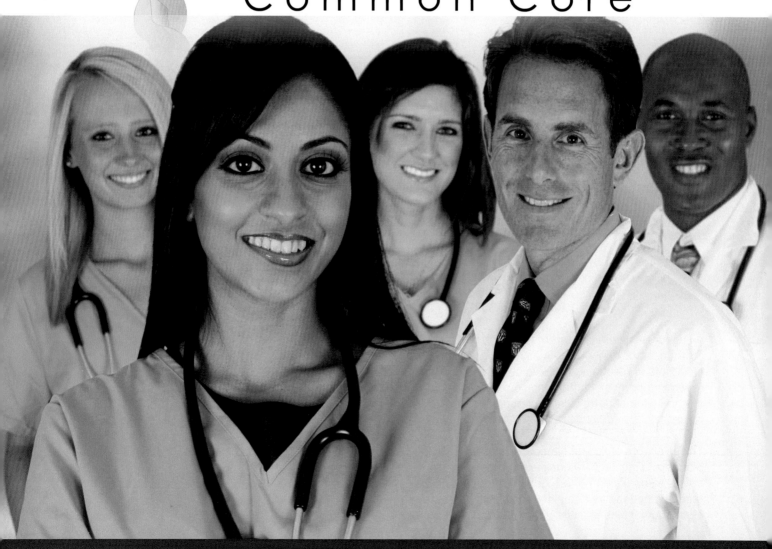

Sabrina Hutton Edmond, M.A. Ed

To order additional copies of this book, contact:
Xlibris
1-888-795-4274
www.Xlibris.com
Orders@Xlibris.com

Medicine
for the
MIND

CHAPTER 1

Introduction to Health Careers

Chapter 1

Unit 1

Introduction to Being a Health Care Worker

History of Health Care

UNIT RATIONALE

Health care has developed and changed throughout history. Knowing the history of health care helps you understand current procedures, practices, and philosophies. The experiences and discoveries of the past led to the advances of today. Today's achievements could not have occurred without the trials and errors of the past. When you understand the primitive beginnings of medicine, you appreciate the advances made during the past 5,000 years.

UNIT OBJECTIVES

When you have completed this unit, you will be able to do the following:

* Match vocabulary words with their correct meanings.

* Identify nine scientists and explain what they contributed to medicine.

* Choose one era in the history of health care and write a paper to explain how health care technology changed.

* Discuss advances in medicine in the twentieth century.

* Research and report on possible advances in medicine for the twenty-first century.

* Explain medical ethics and how it affects health care workers and patients/clients.

* Compare health care in the past with health care in the twentieth and twenty –first centuries.

EARLY BEGINNINGS

Primitive human beings had no electricity, few tools, and poor shelter. Their time was spent protecting themselves against **predators** and finding food. They were **superstitious** and believed that illness and disease were caused by supernatural spirits. In an attempt to heal, tribal doctors performed ceremonies to exorcise evil spirits. They used herbs and plants as medicines. Some of the same medicines are still used today. Here are some examples:

- Digitalis comes from the foxglove plant. Today it is given in pill form, **intravenously**, or by injection. In early times, people chewed the leaves of the foxglove plant to strengthen and slow the heartbeat.

- Quinine comes from the bark of the cinchona tree. It controls fever, relives muscle spasms, and helps prevent malaria.

- Belladonna and atropine are made from the poisonous nightshade plant. They relieve muscle spasm, especially in gastrointestinal (GI) pain.

- Morphine is made from the opium poppy, it relieves severe pain. It is addicting and is used only when nothing else will help.

MEDICINE IN ACIENT TIMES

The Egyptians were the earliest people to keep accurate health records. They were superstitious and called upon the gods to heal them. They also learned to identify certain diseases. They used medicines to heal disease and learned the art of splinting fractures.

The ancient Greeks were the first to study the causes of disease. They kept records on what they observed and what they thought caused illness. The Greeks understood the importance of searching for new information about disease. This research helped eliminate superstition.

During ancient times, religious custom did not allow bodies to be dissected. The father of medicine, Hippocrates(ca. 469-377 B.C.), based his knowledge of anatomy and physiology on **observation** of the external body. He kept careful notes of the signs and symptoms of many diseases. With these records he found that disease was not caused by supernatural forces. Hippocrates wrote the standard of ethics called the Oath of Hippocrates. This standard is the basis for today's medical ethics. Physicians still take this oath.

The Greeks observed and measured the effects of disease. They found that some disease was caused by lack of sanitation. The Romans learned from the Greeks and developed a sanitation system. They brought clean water into their cities by way of aqueducts (waterways). They built sewers to carry off waste. They also built public baths with filtering systems. This was the beginning of public health and sanitation.

The Romans were the first to organize medical care. They sent medical equipment and physicians with their armies to care for wounded soldiers. Roman physicians kept a room in their houses for the ill. This was the beginning of hospitals. Public buildings for the care of the sick were established. Physicians were paid by the Roman government. It is interesting to note that the Roman physician wore a death mask. This mask had a spice-filled beak, which the Romans believed protected them from infection and bad odors.

THE DARK AGES (A.D. 400-800) AND THE MIDDLE AGES (A.D. 800-1400)

When the Roman Empire was conquered by the Huns (nomads from the north), the study of medical science stopped. For a period of 1,000 years, medicine was practiced only in **convents** and **monasteries**. Because the Church believed that life and death were in God's hands, the monks and priests had no interest in how the body functioned. Medication consisted of herbal mixtures, and care was custodial. Monks collected and translated the writings of the Greek and Roman physicians.

Terrible epidemics caused millions of deaths during this period. Bubonic plague (the black death) alone killed 60 million people. Other uncontrolled diseases included smallpox, diphtheria, syphilis, and tuberculosis. Today, these illnesses are not always life threatening. Scientists have discovered vaccines and medications to control these diseases. It is important to remember that some diseases can become epidemic if people are not vaccinated.

THE RENAISSANCE (A.D. 1350-1650)

The Renaissance period saw the rebirth of learning. During this period, new scientific progress began. There were many developments during this period:

- The building of universities and medical schools for research

- The search for new ideas about disease rather than the unquestioning acceptance of disease as the will of God

- The acceptance of **dissection** of the body for study

- The development of the printing press and publishing of books, allowing greater access to knowledge from research

These changes influenced the future of medical science.

THE SIXTEENTH AND SEVENTEENTH CENTURIES

The desire for learning that began during the Renaissance continued through the next two centuries. During this time, several outstanding scientists added new knowledge. Here are some examples:

- Leonardo da Vinci studied and recorded the anatomy of the body

- William Harvey used this knowledge to understand physiology, and he was able to describe the circulation of blood and the pumping of the heart.

- Gabriele Fallopius discovered the fallopian tubes of the female anatomy.

- Bartolommeo Eustachio discovered the tube leading from the ear to the throat(Eustachian tube)

- Antonie van Leeuwenhoek invented the microscope, establishing that there is life smaller than the eye can see. Van Leeuwenhoek scraped his teeth and observed the bacteria that cause tooth decay. Although it was not yet realized, the germs that cause disease were now visible. Unfortunately **quackery**, mass death from childbed fever, and disease continued. The causes of infection and disease were still not understood.

THE EIGHTEENTH CENTURY

Many discoveries were made in the eighteenth century that required a new way of teaching medicine. Students not only attended lectures in the classroom and laboratory, but also observed patients at the bedside. When a patient died, they dissected the body and were able to observe the disease process. This led to a better understanding of the causes of illness and death. The study of physiology continued, and more new discoveries were made:

Rene Laennec invented the **stethoscope**. The first stethoscope was made of wood. It increased the ability to hear the heart and lungs, allowing doctors to determine if disease was present.

Joseph Priestley discovered the element oxygen. He also observed that plants refresh air that has lost its oxygen, making it usable for respiration.

Benjamin Franklin's discoveries affect us in many ways. His discoveries include bifocals, and he found that colds could be passed from person to person.

Edward Jenner discovered a method of vaccination for smallpox. Smallpox killed many people in epidemics. His discovery saved millions of lives. His discovery also led to immunization and to preventive medicine in public health.

THE NINETEENTH AND TWENTIETH CENTURIES

Medicine continued to progress rapidly, and the nineteenth century was the beginning of the organized advancement of medical science. Important events during the nineteenth and twentieth centuries include the following:

- Ignaz Semmelweis identified the cause of childbed fever (puerperal fever). Large numbers of women died from this fever after giving birth. Semmelweis noted that the patients of midwives (women who delivered babies but were not physicians) had fewer deaths. One of the differences in the care given by the physicians and the midwives was that the physicians went to the "dead room," where they dissected dead bodies. These physicians did not wash their hands or change their aprons before they delivered babies. Their hands were dirty, and they infected the women. Semmelweis realized what was happening, but other physicians laughed at him. Eventually, his studies were proved correct by others, and hand washing and cleanliness became an accepted practice. Today, hand washing is still one of the most important ways that we control the spread of infection.

- Louis Pasteur discovered that tiny **microorganisms** were everywhere. Through his experiments and studies, he proved that microorganisms cause disease. Before this discovery, doctors thought that microorganisms were created by disease. He also discovered that heating milk prevented the growth of bacteria. Pasteurization kills bacteria in milk. We still use this method to treat milk today.

- Joseph Lister learned about Pasteur's discovery that microorganisms cause infection. He used carbolic acid on wounds to kill germs that cause infection. He became the first doctor to use an antiseptic during surgery. Using an **antiseptic** during surgery helped prevent infection in the incision.

- Ernst Von Bergmann developed **asepsis**. He knew from Lister's and Pasteur's research that germs caused infections in wounds. He developed a method to keep an area germ-free before and during surgery. This was the beginning of asepsis.

- Robert Koch discovered many disease-causing organisms. He is considered the father of microbiology. He also introduced the importance of cleanliness and sanitation in preventing the spread of disease.

- Wilhelm Rentgen discovered x-rays in 1895. This discovery allowed doctors to see inside the body and helped them discover what was wrong with the patient.

- Paul Ehrlich discovered the effect of medicine on disease-causing microorganisms. His treatment was effective against some microorganisms but was not effective in killing other bacteria. His discoveries brought about the use of chemicals to fight disease. In his search to find a chemical to treat syphilis, he completed 606 experiment, he found a treatment that worked.

Before the nineteenth century, pain was a serious problem. Surgery was performed on patients without **anesthesia**. Early physicians used herbs, hashish, and alcohol to help relieve the pain of surgery. They even choked patients to cause unconsciousness to stop pain. Many patients died from shock and pain. During the nineteenth and twentieth centuries, nitrous oxide (for dental care), eher, and chloroform were discovered. These drugs have the ability to put people into a deep sleep so that they do not experience pain during surgery. The knowledge of asepsis and the ability to prevent pain during surgery are the basis of safe, painless surgery today.

Scientists and physicians learn from the discoveries of the past. They continue to study and research new ways to treat diseases, illness, and injury. Some of the most important discoveries in recent times include the following:

- Gerhard Domagk discovered sulfonamide compounds. These compounds were the first medications effective in killing bacteria. They changed the practice of medicine by killing deadly diseases.

- In 1892 in Russia, Dmitri Ivanovski discovered that some diseases are caused by microorganisms that cannot be seen with a microscope. They are called viruses. These viruses were not studied until the electron microscope was invented in Germany. These are some of the diseases caused by viruses: *Poliomyelitis*Rabies*Measles*Influenza*Chicken pox*German measles*Herpes zoster*Mumps

- Sigmund Freud discovered the conscious and unconscious parts of the mind. He studied the effects of the unconscious mind on the body. He determined that the mind and body work together. This led to an understanding of psychosomatic illness (physical illness caused by emotional conflict). His studies were the basis of psychology and psychiatry.

- Alexander Fleming found that penicillin killed life-threatening bacteria. The discovery of penicillin is considered one of the most important discoveries of the twentieth century. Before penicillin was discovered, people died of illnesses that we consider curable today, including pneumonia, gonorrhea, and blood poisoning.

- Jonas Salk discovered that a dead polio virus would cause immunity to poliomyelitis. This virus paralyzed thousands of adults and children every year. It seemed to attack the most active and athletic people. It was a feared disease, and the discovery of the vaccine saved many people from death or crippling.

- In contrast to Salk's virus, Albert Sabin used a live polio virus vaccine, which is more effective. This vaccine is used today to immunize babies against this dreaded disease.

The discovery of methods to control whooping cough, diphtheria, measles, tetanus, and smallpox saved many lives. These diseases kill unprotected children and adults. It is important for everyone to be immunized. Immunizations are available from doctors, clinics, hospitals, and public health services. Our society is discovering new approaches to medical care every year.

Patients/clients are being taught more about wellness, and they are learning more about self-care. Family and friends are learning patient care skills, including how to perform detailed procedures. Nurses and technicians are visiting patients/clients at home or caring for them in an ambulatory care setting. Just a few years ago, patients were admitted to the hospital for surgery and recovered in the hospital over a period of several days. Today, many patients enter the hospital, have surgery, and are sent home the same day.

People are living longer and are usually healthier. New inventions and procedures have changed medicine as we once knew it. Here are some examples:

- The possibility of eliminating disabling disease through genetic research d

- The ability to transplant organs from a donor to a **recipient**

- The ability to reattach severed body parts

- The use of computers to aid in diagnosis, accurate record keeping, and research

- The ability to use **noninvasive** techniques for diagnosis

- The advancement in caring for the unborn fetus

- The rediscovery and the medical profession's greater acceptance of alternative medicine and complementary medical practice including acupuncture, acupressure, herbal therapy, and healing touch

Every day, science makes new progress. We are living in a time of great advancement and new understanding in medicine. People are living longer, creating a need to better understand geriatric medicine. Frontiers in medical science include hope for treatment and eventually cures for: diabetes, cancer, AIDS, multiple sclerosis, arthritis, and muscular dystrophy.

THE ADVANCEMENT OF NURSING

In the nineteenth century, nursing became an important part of medical care. In 1860, Florence Nightingale (1820-1910) attracted well-educated, dedicated women to the Nightingale School of Nursing. The graduates from this school raised the standards of nursing, and nursing became a respectable profession. Before this, nursing was considered unsuitable for a respectable lady. The people giving care to patients were among the lowest in society-"too old, too weak, too drunken, too dirty, or too bad to do anything else."

Florence Nightingale came from a cultured, middle-class family who opposed her interest in caring for the ill. However, she convinced her father to give her money to live, and she gained experience by volunteering in hospitals. During the Crimean War, she took a group of 38 women to care for soldiers dying from cholera. More soldiers were dying from cholera than from war injuries. She became a legend while she was there because of her dedication to nursing. After the war she devoted much of her life to preparing reports on the need for better sanitation and construction and management of hospitals. Her primary goal was to gain effective training for nurses. The public

established a Nightingale fund to pay for the training protection, and living costs of nurses. This was established in recognition of her services to the military during the Crimean War. She also designed a hospital ward that improved the environment and care of the patients. Prior to this time, patients were crowded into small areas that were often dirty. The ward that she designed allowed for a limited number of beds, permitted circulation of air, had windows on three sides, and was clean.

During this time, Clara Barton (1821-1912) served as a volunteer nurse in the American Civil War. After the war, she established a bureau of records to help search for missing men. She also assisted in the organization of military hospitals in Europe during the Franco-Prussian War. These experiences led her to establish the American Red Cross. Another step forward in the field of nursing was contributed by Lillian Wald (1867-1940). She was an American public health nurse and social reformer. She established the Henry Street Settlement in New York

to homes of the poor. This led to the Visiting Nurse Service of New York. Today, visiting nurse services are found in most communities.

PATIENT CARE TODAY

Nursing care has changed many times throughout the years. Patients have been cared for by teams that included a registered nurse as a team leader, a licensed vocational nurse or practical nurse (LVN/LPN) as a medication nurse, and a nursing assistant who provided personal care. In primary care nursing, which followed team nursing, all patient care was provided by a registered nurse. Today, unlicensed assistive caregivers are part of the patient caregiver team. There are many titles and new job descriptions for these positions, including clinical partner, service partner, nurse extender, health care assistant, and patient care assistant. These new positions extend the role of entry-level employees. The nurse assistant performs additional tasks, such as phlebotomy and recording and electrocardiogram (EKG). Employees from departments other than nursing learn patient care skills. Environmental service workers and food service workers may help with serving food and providing some routine patient care. The registered nurse delegates patient care tasks according to the training and expertise of the assistive personnel.

A LOOK BACK AND AN OVERIVEW OF THE FUTURE

In the twentieth century, medicine is making great strides in improving health care. During this century, we experienced many changes, including these:

Antibiotics for bacterial diseases

Improved life expectancy

Organ transplants

Healthier hearts (reduced smoking, better diets)

Dentistry without pain

Childhood immunizations

Noninvasive diagnosis with computers (CAT, MRI)

End of smallpox

Childhood immunizations

New understanding of DNA and genetics

Control of diabetes

Decline in polio

The future of medicine holds many promises for better health. Current and future research will provide us with many new advances, including these:

Cure for AIDS

Decrease in the cases of malaria, influenza, leprosy, and African sleeping sickness

Cure for genetically transferred diseases (e.g. Tay-Sachs, muscular dystrophy, multiple sclerosis, cerebral palsy, Alzheimer's, lupus)

Improved treatment for arthritis and the common cold

Isolation of the gene that causes depression

Use of electronics to allow disabled persons to walk

Nutritional therapy to decrease the number of cases of schizophrenia

MEDICAL ETHICS

Advancement in medicine creates new problems. How will the recipient of an organ be chosen? Who will be allowed to receive experimental drugs? How will the creation of in vitro embryos be ethically managed? Is it ethical to provide continuing confidentiality about AIDS patients, or should they be required to report their condition? Does a terminally ill patient have the right to assisted death (euthanasia)? There are many questions now, and there will be more questions in the future as health care changes.

SUMMARY

You have learned that the science of health care has grown and developed over the last 5,000 years. These changes increased the average life expectancy. Our standards of living improved with the progress of medical science. The dedication of the many scientists discussed in this unit is responsible for the improvements in health care that we enjoy today. Their research is the foundation of the high technology that is developing in medicine.

UNIT 2

Health Care Providers

UNIT RATIONAL

It is the responsibility of every health care worker to help patients/clients solve their health problems. Since the health care industry has many delivery systems, it is important for future health care workers to be aware of health care agencies and facilities, their delivery systems, their organization, and some of their major services. When you understand how health care facilities and agencies serve the public, you will become a resource person for members of your community.

UNIT OBJECTIVES

When you have completed this unit, you will be able to do the following:

- Match vocabulary words with their correct meanings.

- Write a report on a volunteer agency.

- Define managed care.

- Define ambulatory care.

- Evaluate how managed care and ambulatory care meet the needs of the changing health care system.

- List six types of outpatient care and the type of treatment given.

- Define wellness and preventive care

- Contrast the current trends with health care in the twentieth century.

- Fill in an organizational chart.

- Give two reasons why the organization of health care facilities is important.

- Explain a chain of command.

- List and define the major services in health care.

- Identify two departments in each major service.

TYPES OF HEALTH CARE PROVIDERS

There are several facilities and agencies that provide medical care. Some are familiar, and others will be new to you. The following of descriptions will help you understand the differences among the many providers of medical care.

CHAPTER 2

METRIC APOTHECARY & HOUSEHOLD CONVERSIONS

Chapter 2

Metric, Apothecary, and Household Conversions

Review the equivalents given Table 7.1

Table 7.1

Equivalents

Household	Apothecary	Metric
	Weight	
	1 gr=	60mg
	60 gr =	1 3 (dram)
	8 3 =	1 3 (ounce)
	Liquid	
15-16gtt (drops)	$\simeq$ 15-16 m x (minim)	1 ml (cc)
1 tsp	$\simeq$ 1 3	4-5 ml
1 tbsp	$\simeq$ 4 3	15-16 ml
	8 3 = 3	30 ml
1 teacup	= 6 3	180 ml
1 glass	= 8 3	240 ml
1 pt	= 16 3	500 ml
2 pt = 1 qt	= 32 3	1000 ml
4 qt = 1 gal	= 128 3	

To convert one measurement system to another use ratio-proportion principles. Each problem must begin with the known equivalent.

Example: To change ¼ gr to mg, you must know that 60 mg = 1 gr.

Known equivalent

60 mg/= X mg

1 gr /= ¼ gr

Cross multiply to solve for x.

X= 60 X ¼

X= 60/4

X= **15** mg

....

....

....

....

....

Example: Change 10mg to gr

Known equivalent 60 mg = 10mg

1 gr = X gr

60 X= 10

X = 10/60

X = 1/6 gr

When converting between the metric and apothecary systems of measurement we usually use the equivalent 60 mg = 1 gr. However, there are times when approximate equivalents appear in problems. In these instances do not compute the answer using 60 mg = 1 gr. Just recognize the approximate equivalent and write the appropriate answer.

Approximate Equivalents

50 mg ~ ¾ gr	300 mg ~ 5 gr
100 mg ~ 1 ½ gr	500 mg~ 7 ½ gr
200 mg ~ 3 gr	1000 mg ~ 15gr
250 mg ~ 3 ¾	

Example: The order is written give Seconal gr 1 ½. How many milligrams is this? 100 mg. If the problem had been worked with 60 mg = 1 gr, the answer derived would have been 90. That is incorrect.

Try another. Give 50 mg of Demerol. How many grains is this? ¾ gr

You must know the approximate equivalent table as well as the other measurement tables.

PRACTICE PROBLEMS

1. 15 gr = mg

2. 19 ml = m_2

3. 0.25 Gm =_gr=_mg

4. 15 mg =_gr

5. 1/8 gr = mg

6. 39 kg =_lb

7. 3 iv = tsp

8. 15 ml = 3

9. ½ gal = ml = qtr.

10. 250 ml = pt.

11. 16 ml 3 = Tbsp.

12. 750 mg = gr

13. 750 ml = qtr.

14. 3 Gm =gr =mg

15. 1/150 gr = mg

16. 0.6 mg = gr =Gm

17. 400 Gm= mg=gr

18. 1/200 gr = mg

19. 3 ss = ml

20. 60 ml = ____ tsp

21. 64 3 = ____ L

22. 45 ml = ____ 3

23. 79 kg = ____ lb.

24. 250 mg = ____ gr

25. 12 ml = ____ gtt

26. 0.1 mg = ____ gr

27. 15 ml = ____ 3

28. 1/60 gr = ____ mg = ____ Gm

29. 60 ml = ____ Tbsp.

30. 4 teacups = ____ ml

31. 360 ml = ____ glasses

32. 16 3 = ____ ml

33. 1/600 gr = ____ mg = ____ Gm

34. 3500 ml = ____ pt.

35. 2.5 L = ____ qtr.

36. 6 qtr. = ____ ml

37. 150 mg = ____ gr

38. 10 kg = ____ lb.

Unit 2

Comprehensive Test

Calculate the following metric, apothecary, and household problems.

1. 216 ml = _____ L = _____ cc

2. 804 l = _____ Klo

3. 250 cc = _____ ml = _____ L

4. 4854 ml = _____ Klo

5. 6.328 Klo = _____ L = _____ ml

6. 21.60 ml = _____ L

7. 340 L = _____ cc = _____ Klo

8. 242.4 Klo = _____ cc

9. 1755 cc = _____ L = _____ ml

10. 310.7 L = _____ Klo

11. 4240 cc = _____ Klo = _____ L

12. 45.63 ml = _____ cc

13. 510 Klo = _____ ml = _____ L

14. 1320 L = _____ ml

15. 21, 014 cc = _____ Klo = _____ ml

16. 90,009 L = _____ Klo

17. 4816 ml = _____ L = _____ cc

18. 5212 mcg = _____ Gm

19. 14,000 mcg = _____ mg

CHAPTER 3

ORAL MEDICATIONS

Chapter 3

Oral Medications

Generally, oral medications come in the dosage ordered. There are times, however, when the nurse must calculate the number or portion of tablets or the amount of liquid to administer. The first step in solving these problems will be to make sure the desired dosage (D) and the dosage on hand (H) are in the same unit of measurement.

Example: In order to administer gr 1/8 of a drug which is available in 15 mg tablets you must convert 1/8 gr to mg or 15 mg to gr.

(a) 60 mg = X mg

  1 gr = 1/8 gr

  X = 60 X 1/8

  X= 60/8

  X= 7.5 mg

(b) 60 mg = 15 mg

  1 gr = X gr

  60X= 15

  X= 15/60

  X= ¼ gr

The next step is to use the formula.

D/H = Amount to give Dosage desired/dosage on hand= amount to give

Example:

Gr 1/8 =4= 1

Gr ¼ =8= 2 = tablet

Remember it is possible to give part of a scored tablet; however, it is not possible to give part of a capsule.

Example: Give 4 mg of a drug which comes in 2 mg tablets.

Desired dosage 4 mg

Dosage on hand = 2 mg = 2 tablets

To give a drug which comes in a liquid form, the formula to use is:

D/H X Amount of Liquid= Amount to give

Example: Give 125 mg of liquid medication which comes 250 mg per 5 ml.

125
250 X 5

1
2 X 5 = 2.5 ml

Points to remember:

Step one: **Convert measurement system if necessary.**
Step two: **Formula to solve for drug dosage**

Desired dosage
Dose on hand = Amount to give

Desired dosage
Dose on hand X Amount of liquid = Amount to give

PRACTICE PROBLEMS

1. Ordered: Ampicillin 0.25 Gm po q 6 hr.
   On hand: Ampicillin 125 mg po   Give _____ cap

2. Ordered: Diamox 500 mg po qd
   On hand: Diamox 125 mg po   Give _____ tab

3. Ordered: Chloral Hydrate gr viiss po H.S.
   On hand: Chloral Hydrate 500 mg po   Give _____ cap

4. Ordered: Polycillin 250 mg po q4 hr.
   On hand: Polycillin 100 mg per 5 ml   Give _____ ml

5. Ordered: Azo Gantrsin 500 mg po qid
   On hand: Azo Gantrisin 1 Gm po   Give _____ tab

6. Ordered: Zyloprim 100 mg po tid
   On hand: Zyloprim 25 mg po   Give _____ tab

7. Ordered: Benadryl gr ss po q 8 hr.
   On hand: Benadryl 15 mg po   Give _____ cap

8. Ordered: Maalox 3 ss po q 4 hr
    On hand: Maalox liquid   Give _____ ml

9. Ordered: Antivert 25 mg pot id
    On hand: Antivert 10 mg po   Give _____ tab

10. Ordered: Elix Phenobarbital 15 mg po q 8 hr.
    On hand: Elix Phenobarbital 20 mg/5 ml   Give _____ ml

11. Ordered: Inderal 80 mg po Bid
    On hand: Inderal 20 mg po   Give _____ tab

12. Ordered: Lanoxin 0.25 mg po qd
    On hand: Lanoxin 0.125 mg po   Give _____ tab

13. Ordered: Benadryl 25 mg pot id
    On hand: Benadryl 12.5 mg/5 ml po   Give _____ ml

14. Ordered: Valium gr 1/60 po q 4 hr.
    On hand: Valium 2 mg po   Give _____ tab

15. Ordered: Chloral Hydrate 250 mg po H.S.
    On hand: Chloral Hydrate gr viiss/5 ml po   Give _____ ml

16. Ordered: Nilstat 300,000 U pot id
    On hand: Nilstat 100,000 U/ml po   Give _____ ml

17. Ordered: Catapres 0.1 mg po H.S.
    On hand: Catapres gr 1/300 po   Give _____ tab

18. Ordered: Thyroid gr 1/300 po qd
    On hand: Thyroid 0.2 mg po   Give _____ tab

19. Ordered: Ampicillin 1 Gm po q 8 hr.
    On hand: Ampicillin gr 3 ¾ po   Give _____ cap

20. Ordered: Nembutal gr iss po H.S.
    On hand: Nembutal 100 mg po   Give _____ cap

21. Ordered: Inderal gr 2/3 po Bid
    On hand: Inderal 20 mg po   Give _____ cap

22. Ordered: Potassium Chloride 15 m Eq pot id
    On hand: Potassium Chloride 20 m Eq/10 ml po   Give _____ ml

23. Ordered: Phenergan 12.5 mg pot id
    On hand: Phenergan 25 mg po   Give _____ tab

24. Ordered: Persantine 25 mg pot id
    On hand: Persantine gr 1/6 po   Give _____ tab

25. Ordered: Tagamet 300 mg po q 6 hr.
    On hand: Tagamet gr v po   Give _____ tab

26. Ordered: Dilaudid gr 1/16 po q 4 hr. PRN
    On hand: Dilaudid gr 1/32 po   Give _____ tab

27. Ordered: Nitroglycerine gr 1/200 po PRN
    On hand: Nitroglycerine 0.16 mg po   Give _____ tab

28. Ordered: Elavil 75 mg po H.S.
    On hand: Elavil 25 mg po   Give _____ tab

29. Ordered: Polycillin 500,000 U po qid
    On hand: Polycillin 4,000,000 U/10 ml po   Give _____ ml

30. Ordered: Aspirin 0.16 Gm po q 4 hr
    On hand: Aspirin 300 mg po   Give _____ tab

31. Ordered: Doxidan 300 mg po qd
    On hand: Doxidan 0.5 Gm/10 ml po   Give _____ ml

32. Ordered: Mylanta 3ss po q 4 hr.
    On hand: Mylanta liquid   Give _____ ml

33. Ordered: Elix Phenobarbital gr ss po H.S.
    On hand: Elix Phenobarbibtal 100 mg/10 ml   Give _____ ml

34. Ordered: Lasix 40 mg po qd
    On hand: Lasix gr 1/6 po   Give _____ tab

35. Ordered: Clinoril 125 mg po Bidd
    On hand: Clinoril 0.5 Gm po   Give _____ tab

36. Ordered: Elix Lanoxin 0.025 mg po qd
    On hand: Elix lanoxin 0.05 mg/5 ml po   Give _____ ml

37. Ordered: Catapres 0.4 mg po qd
    On hand: Catapres gr 1/150 po   Give _____ tab

38. Ordered: Flexeril 20 mg pot id
   On hand: Flexeril gr 1/6 po   Give _____ tab

39. Ordered: ASA sup gr x q 4 hr. PRN
   On hand: ASA sup 300 mg   Give _____ sup

40. Ordered: Dilantin 100 mg pot id
   On hand: Dilantin gr iss po   Give _____ cap

41. Give Clinoril 5 gr from a bottle labeled Clinoril 150 mg. Give _____ tab

42. In order to administer Morphine Sulfate 10 mg from tablets labeled M.S. gr 1/6 you would give how many tablets? _____ Tab

43. The order reads Elix Phenobarbital 20 mg. Available is a bottle labeled Elix Phenobarbital gr ¼ per 5 ml. You would give _____ ml?

44. Ordered is Potassium Chloride 45 mEq po. The label reads KCl 15 mEq/5 ml. You would give _____ ml? _____ 3?

45. In giving Atropine gr 1/500 you would be giving _____ mg?

46. The written order is Valium 2.5 mg. The tablets available are labeled gr 1/6. How many tablets would you give? _____ Tab

47. Give Inderal 0.24 mg po from a solution labeled Inderal 2 mg per 10 ml. _____ ml

48. The order reads Benadryl 50 mg po. The solution is labeled Benadryl 12.5 mg/5 ml. You would give _____ ml? _____ 3?

CHAPTER 4

PARENTERAL DOSAGES

Chapter 4
Parenteral Dosages

Parenteral medications are those given by injection. The most common parenteral routes used by nurses are intradermal, subcutaneous, intramuscular (or "IM"), and intravenous (or "IV").

Medications given parenterally must be in liquid form to be injected. Some of these medications are prepared as liquids by the pharmaceutical companies and placed into vials or ampules. The label states the amount of medication in a given amount of liquid. Other medications are not stable as liquids and must be packaged as powders. The powdered medications come in vials and must be mixed with sterile water or normal saline prior to injection. The label on the vial or the package insert will tell the amount and type of solution to be mixed with the powder. Parenteral medications may be dispensed in micrograms, milligrams, grams, milliequivalents, and in units. Syringes are used to administer parenteral medications. Commonly used are the 3 cc syringe, the 1 cc or tuberculin syringe, and the insulin syringe.

Examples of different preparations of parenteral medications

(A)

_____

_____

_____

(B)

_____

_____

_____

(C)

_____

_____

_____

The markings in the 3 cc syringe are measured in cc's, in tenths of a cc, and in minims.

_____

_____

_____

Three cc syringe

The markings on the tuberculin or 1 cc syringe are measured in hundredths and tenths of a cc and in minims.

_____

_____

_____

Tuberculin (1 cc) syringe

There are two types of insulin syringes. One is a 1 cc syringe marked off in 100 units. The other is a ½ cc syringe which is marked off in 50 units.

Insulin (1 cc) syringe

_____

_____

_____

Insulin (1/2 cc) syringe

After calculating the amount of medication to be administered, the medication is drawn into the proper syringe and measured as is illustrated.

_____

_____

_____

Syringe filled with 2 cc of medication

Parenteral dosage problems can be solved by the ratio and proportion method or by using the formula D/H X Amount. Remember that when using the formula, D and H must be in the same system. We will solve the following problem using both methods.

_____

Example: Give Ampicillin 500 mg from a vial labeled Ampicillin 250 mg per 5 cc.

Using the ratio and proportion method, proceed as follows:

$$250 \text{ mg}: 5 \text{ cc}: 500 \text{mg}: X \text{ cc}$$
$$250 \text{ X cc} = 2500$$

$$\frac{250 \text{ X cc}}{250} = \frac{2500}{250}$$

$$X = \mathbf{10 \text{ cc}}$$

To use the formula D/H X Amount of liquid, set up the problem as:

$$\frac{500 \text{ mg}}{250 \text{ mg}} \times 5 \text{ cc} = \mathbf{10cc}$$

Example: try another problem. The order is for Procaine Penicillin G 150,000 units. The drug is available as 300,000 units/ml. Use the formula D/H X Amount –the order is the desired dosage.

$$\frac{150,000 \text{ U}}{300,000 \text{ U}} \times 1 \text{ ml} = \mathbf{0.5 \text{ ml}}$$

RX List

The Internet drug index

Based upon more than 3 billion prescriptions: Data furnished by NDC Health

Brand Name	Manufacturer	Generic Name
Hydrocodone w/APAP*	Various**	Hydrocodone w/APAP
Lipitor	Pfizer Us Pharm	Atorvastatin
Synthroid	Abbott	Levothyroxine
Atenolol	Various	Atenolol
Zithromax	Pfizer US Pharm	Azithromycin
Amoxicillin	Various	Amoxicillin
Furosemide	Various	Furosemide
Hydrochlorothiazide	Various	Hydrochlorothiazide
Norvasc	Pfizer US Pharm	Amlodipine
Lisinopril	Various	Lisinopril
Alprazolam	Various	Alprazolam
Zoloft	Pfizer US Pharm	Amlodipine
Albuterol Aerosol	Various	Albuterol

Toprol-XL	AstraZeneca	Metoprolol
Zocor	MSD	Simvastatin
Premarin	Wyeth Pharm	Conjugated Estrogens
Prevacid	Tap Pharm	Lansoprazole
Zyrtec	Pfizer US Pharm	Cetirizine
Ibuprofen	Various	Ibuprofen
Levoxyl	Monarch Pharm	Levothyroxine
Propoxyphene N/APAP	Various	Propoxyphene N/APAP
Triamterene/HCTZ	Various	Traimterene/HCTZ
Celebrex	Pharmacia Upjohn	Celecoxib
Ambien	Sanofi	Zolpidem
Cyclobenzaprine	Various	Cyclobenzaprine
Glucotrol XL	Pfizer US Pharm	Glipizide
Diflucan	Pfizer US Pharm	Fluconazole
Verapamil	Various	Verapamil
Bextra	Pharmacia Upjohn	Valdecoxib
Penicillin VK	Various	Penicillin VK
Cozaar	MSD	Losartan
Actos	Takeda	Pioglitazone
Trazodone	Various	Trazodone
Glyburide	Various	Glyburide
Naproxen	Various	Naproxen
Diovan HCT	Novartis	Valsartan/ HCTZ
Coumadin	BMS	Warfarin
Ortho Evra	Ortho	Norelgestromin/Ethinyl
Avandia	GlaxoSmithKline	Rosigiltazone maleate
Paxil CR	GlaxoSmithKline	Paroxetine
Risperdal	Janssen	Risperidone
Flomax	Abbott	Tamsulosin
Aciphex	Eisai	Rabeprazole
Digitek	Bertek	Digoxin
Cipro	Bayer	Ciproflaxacin
Nasonex	Schering	Mometasone
Oxycondone/APAP	Mallinkrt Pharm	Oxycodone/APAP
Glucophage XR	BMS Primary Care	Metformin
Lotensin	Novartis	Benazepril
Evista	Lilly	Raloxifene
Zyprexa	Lilly	Olanzapine
Diltiazem HCl	Various	Diltiazem
Allegra-D	Aventis	Fexofenadine

Clonidine	Mylan	Clonidine
Lanoxin	GlaxoSmithKline	Digoxin
Hyzaar	MSD	Losartan/HCTZ
Amoxil	GlaxoSmithKline	Digoxin
Actonel	P & G	Risedronate
Oxycontin	Purdue	Oxycodone
Xalatan	Teva	Trimeth/Sulfameth
Xalatan	Pharmacia Upjohn	Latanoprost
Tricor	Abbott	Fenofibrate
Macrobid	P& G Pharm	Nitrofurantoin
Temazepam	Mylan	Temazepam
Doxycycline Hyclate	Watson	Doxycycline
Imitrex	GlaxoSmithKline	Sumatriptan
Necon	Watson	Ethinyl Estradiol
Klor-Con	Upsher-Smith	Potassium Chloride
Allopurinol	Mylan	Allopurinol
Dilantin	Pfizer Pharm	Phenytoin
SMZ-TMP	Mutual	Trimeth/Sulfameth
Microgestin Fe	Watson	Norethindrone
Humalog	Lilly	Insulin Lispro
Cefzil	BMS Primary Care	Cefprozil
Duragesic	Janssen	Fentanyl
Bactroban	GlaxoSmithKline	Mupirocin
Patanol	Alcon	Olopatadine
Humulin 70/30	Lilly	Human Insulin 70/30
Aricept	Eisai	Donepezil
Miralax	Braintree	PEG 3350
Aviane	Barr	Levonorgestrel
Zyrtec-D	Pfizer US Pharm	Cetirizine
Ditropan XL	McNeil	Oxybutynin
Biaxin	Abbott	Clarithromycin
Ciprofloxacin	Barr	Ciprofloxacin
Niaspan	Koss Pharm	Niacin
Strattera	Lilly	Atomoxetine
Inderal LA	Wyeth Pharm	Propanolol
Elidel	Novartis	Pimecrolimus
Pulmicort	AstraZeneca	Budesonide
Trivora-28	Watson	Levonorgestrel
Albuterol	Warrick	Albuterol
Nifedipine ER	Barr	Nifedipine

Methylprednisolone	Barr	Methylprednisolone
Tussionex	Celtech Pharm	Hydrocodone
Mobic	Abbott	Meloxicam
Timolol	Falcon Pharm	Timolol
Atacand	AstraZeneca	Candesartan
Phenytoin	Mylan	Phenytoin
Alphagan P	Allergan	Brimonidine
Avelox	Bayer	Moxifloxacin
Clotrimazole/Betamethasone	Bayer	Moxifloacin
Triamcinolone	Fougera	Triamcinolone
Lescol XL	Novartis	Fluvastatin
Miacalcin	Novartis	Calcitonin
Ortho-Novum	Ortho-McNeil	Norethindrone
Plendil	AstraZeneca	Felodipine
Promethazine/Codeine	Alpharma US	Promethazine/Codeine
Nitroquick	Ethex	Nitroglycerin
Spironolactone	Mylan	Spironolactone
Terazosin	Sandoz	Terazosin
Proscar	MSD	Finasteride
Avalide	BMS Primarycare	Irbesartan/HCTZ
Kariva	Barr	Desogestrel
Low-Ogestrel	Watson	Norgestrel
Tobradex	Alcon	Tobramycin
Remeron	Organon	Mirtazapine
Roxicet	Roxane	Oxycodone
Percocet	Endo	Oxycodone
Atrovent	Bi	Ipratropium
Propranolol	Pilva	Propranolol
Nifediac CC	Teva	Nifedipine
Apri	Barr	Desogestrel

CHAPTER 5

HOSPITAL EQUIPMENT USED IN DOSAGES MEASURMENT

Chapter 5

Hospital Equipment Used In Dosage Measurement

Objectives

- Upon mastery, you will be able to measure correctly the prescribed dosages that you calculate. To accomplish this, you will also be able to:

- Recognize and select the appropriate utensil for the drug, dosage, and method of administration ordered.

Read and interpret the calibrations of each utensil presented.

Now that you are familiar with the systems of measurement used in the calculation of medicines, let's take a look at the common utensils used to measure the correct dosage. In this section you will learn to recognize and read the calibrations of a medicine cup, a calibrated dropper, a regular 3-cc syringe, a prefilled syringe, a standard U-100 insulin syringe, a LO-DOSE U-100 insulin syringe, and a tuberculin syringe.

Oral Administration

Medicine Cup

Below shows the 30-millilter or 1-ounce medicine cup that is used to measure most liquids for oral administration. Two views are presented to show all of the scales. Notice that the approximate equivalents of the metric, apothecaries', and household systems of measurement are indicated on the cup. You can see that 30 milliliters equal 1 ounce, 5 milliliters equal 1 teaspoon, and so forth. Look at the calibrations. Milliliters are marked in units of 5, teaspoons are marked in units of ½ to 1, drams are marked in units of 1 and 2, and ounces are marked in units of 1/8 to ¼.

Above is the medicine cup with approximate equivalent measures

(A)

_____

_____

_____

(B)

_____

_____

_____

Calibrated Dropper

Shows the calibrated dropper which is used to administer some small quantities. A dropper is used when giving medicine to children and when adding small amounts of liquid to water or juice. Eye and ear medications are also dispensed from a squeeze-drop bottle. The amount of the drop varies according to the diameter of the dropper. For this reason, the dropper usually accompanies the medicine and is calibrated according to the way the drug is ordered. The calibrations are usually given in milliliters, cubic centimeters, or drops.

Pediatric Oral Devices

Various types of calibrated equipment are available to administer oral medications to children. (B) demonstrates several of these special devices.

Parenteral Administration

The term parenteral is used to designate routes of administration other than oral. However, in this text, parenteral always means injection routes.

3-cc Syringe

Below shows the barrel of a regular 3-cc syringe. Look closely at the metric scale which is calibrated in cubic centimeters (cc) for each tenth (0.1) of a cubic centimeter. Each ½ cubic centimeter is marked up to 3 cubic centimeters. The apothecaries' scale is calibrated in minims. You may disregard this scale, since it is becoming obsolete. It will not be used for the measurement of dosages. Standard drug dosages are to be rounded to the nearest tenth (0.1) of a cc or mL and measured on the cc scale.

Example: 1.25 cc is rounded to 1.3 cc. Notice that the arrow in (C) identifies 1.3 cc.

(C)

_____

_____

_____

(D) 3 cc syringe with needle unit

_____

_____

_____

(D) is a 3-cc syringe assembled with needle unit. The black rubber tip of the suction plunger is visible. This plunger withdraws the medicine from the storage container. The calibrations are read from the top black ring, NOT the raised middle section and NOT the bottom ring. Notice that the plunger measures 2 cc.

Prefilled Syringe

(E) is an example of a prefilled, single-dose syringe. Such syringes contain the usual single dose of a medication and are to be used once and discarded. If you are to give less than the full single dose of a drug provided in a prefilled, single dose syringe, you should discard the extra amount before injecting the patient.

Example: The drug order prescribes 7.5 mg of Valium to be administered to a patient. You have a prefilled, single-dose syringe of Valium containing 10 mg per 2 ml of solution (as in E). You would discard 2.5 mg (0.5 mL) of the drug solution; then, 7.5 mg would be remaining in the syringe.

(E) Prefilled, single-dose syringe

_____

_____

_____

1. (a)

_____

_____

_____

1. (b)

_____

_____

_____

(a)Tubex ® closed injection system and (b) Carpuject ® injection system is used only once and discarded. The medication contained in the cartridge is measured and supplied in the usual single dose. However, if the drug order is for less than the full single dose, you should discard the extra amount before injecting the patient. Another disposable system, the Carpuject ®, is shown in (b).

Note: Most syringes are marked in cubic centimeters (cc), whereas most drugs are prepared and labeled with the strength given per milliliter (mL). Remember that the cubic centimeter and milliliter are equivalent measurements in dosage calculations.

Insulin Syringe

2 (a) shows a standard U-100 insulin syringe. This syringe is to be used for the measurement and administration of U-100 insulin only. Insulin should not be measured in any other type of syringe except in an emergency when insulin syringes are not available. The syringe is calibrated in units (U), for a total of 100 units per 1 cc or 1 mL. The plunger in 2 (a) shows a U-100 LO-DOSE ® insulin syringe. The enlarged scale is easier to read and is calibrated for each 1 unit (U) up to 50 units per ½ (0.5) cc. Every 5 units are marked. The plunger in 2(b) demonstrates the measurement of 19 units.

2 (a)

_____

_____

_____

2(b)

_____

_____

_____

3 (a)

_____

_____

_____

3 (b)

_____

_____

_____

Tuberculin Syringe

1(a) shows the 1 cc tuberculin syringe. 1(b) shows the ½ cc (0.5 mL) tuberculin syringe. This syringe should be used when a small dose of a drug must be measured.

_____

_____

_____

1(a) tuberculin syringe

_____

_____

_____

1(b) ½ cc tuberculin syringe

_____

_____

_____

Practice Problems—Chapter 5

1. In the U-100 insulin syringe, 100 u = _____ cc.

2. The tuberculin syringe is calibrated in of _____ cc.

3. Can you measure 1.25 cc in a single tuberculin syringe? Explain.

_____

_____

4. How would you measure 1.33 mL in a 3-cc syringe?

_____

5. The medicine cup has a _____ capacity.

6. To administer 0.52 cc to a child, select a _____ syringe.

7. 75 U of U-100 insulin equals _____ cc.

8. All droppers are calibrated to deliver a standardized drop of equal amounts. (True) (False)

9. The prefilled syringe is a multiple-dose system. (True) (False)

10. Insulin should be measured in an insulin syringe only, except in an emergency when no insulin syringes are available. (True) (False)

Draw an arrow to indicate the calibration that corresponds to the dose to be administered.

11. Administer 0.45 cc

_____

_____

_____

12. Administer 80 U

_____

_____

_____

USE U-100 ONLY

13. Administer 3 iii

_____

_____

_____

14. Administer 2.4 cc

_____

_____

_____

15. Administer 1.1 cc

_____

_____

_____

CHAPTER 6

MEASURING VITAL SIGNS

Chapter 6

Measuring Vital Signs

Unit 1: Temperature, Pulse, and Respiration

UNIT RATIONALE

Important indicators of your patient's/client's health status are known as vital signs. Vital signs give you information about breathing, body temperature, and the heart. They are a good indication of how well the body systems are functioning. As a health care worker, you need to observe patients whenever you are near them. Your knowledge of vital signs and how to measure them helps you know when to report that a patient is having problems.

UNIT OBJECTIVES

When you have completed this unit, you will be able to do the following:

- Match vocabulary words with their correct meanings.

- Define vital signs

- List fourteen factors that influence body temperature.

- Name the most common site at which to measure a temperature.

- Match the normal temperature to the site where it is measured.

- Measure temperature with a glass thermometer.

- Demonstrate how to measure oral, rectal, and axillary temperature.

- Define pulse.

- Explain pulse oximetry.

- Identify sites where pulse may be counted.

- Identify a normal adult pulse rate and a common method for counting a pulse.

- List six factors that influence the pulse rate.

- Demonstrate counting and recording a radial pulse accurately.

- Recognize two parts of a respiration.

- Relate types of abnormal respirations to their correct name.

- Select eight factors that affect respiration.

- Explain the importance of not being obvious when counting respirations.

- Demonstrate how to count and record respirations accurately.

- Explain the importance of each vital sign.

INTRODUCTION TO VITAL SIGNS

Vital signs include body temperature, pulse, respiration rates, and **blood pressure**. Vital signs are the indicators that tell you how the body is functioning. Pulse oximetry is another important indicator of body functioning. When vital signs are within normal limits, the body is considered to be in homeostasis. When the vital signs are not within normal limits, it is an indication that something is wrong. It is important to be accurate when you measure vital signs and to record the results very carefully and accurately. Other health care workers depend on this information when making decisions about the patient's treatment. In this unit, you learn how to measure body temperature and count the pulse rate and respiratory rate. Together these measurements are referred to as **TPR**.

TEMPERATURE

Temperature is the measure of body heat. Heat is produced in the body by the muscles and glands and by the **oxidation** of food. Heat is lost from the body by respiration, perspiration, and **excretion**. The balance between the heat produced and the heat lost is the body temperature. Table 11.1 shows the factors that influence temperature.

Thermometers

The thermometer is the instrument used to measure temperature. There are several types of thermometers: glass thermometers, aural thermometers, chemically treated paper or plastic thermometers, and electronic/digital thermometers.

GLASS THERMOMETER (CLINICAL/MERCURY)

A glass thermometer is a hollow glass tube with **calibration** lines on it. At one end of the thermometer is a bulb that is filled with mercury. The mercury is heat sensitive and rises up the hollow tube when exposed to hear. This enables you to read the patient's/client's temperature. There are two types of tips or bulbs on glass thermometers. (Figure 1.1)

AURAL THERMOMETERS

A tympanic membrane sensor measures body temperature. It is accurate, easy to use, and safe. It is especially effective for babies and children.

Table 1.1

Factors that Influence Temperature	
Increase Temperature	**Decrease Temperature**
Exercise	Sleep
Digestion of food	Fasting
Increased environmental temperature	Exposure to cold
Illness	Certain illness
Infection	Decreased muscle activity
Excitement	Mouth breathing
Anxiety	Depression

USING AN ELECTRONIC THERMOMETER

Rationale

As a health care worker it is important to monitor the patient's physical status. One way to determine this status is by measuring the patient's body temperature. There are many different kinds of thermometers. This procedure explains how to use an electronic thermometer to measure body temperature.

Alert: Follow Standard Precautions

1. Wash hands.

2. Assemble equipment.

    a. Plastic thermometer covers

    b. Electronic thermometer with appropriate probe (blue for oral, red for rectal)

3. Identify patient/client.

4. Explain procedure to patient.

5. Place plastic thermometer cover over probe.

6. Insert probe in proper position to measure body temperature (blue-tipped probe under tongue or in axilla, red-tipped probe in rectum).

7. Hold probe in place for 15 seconds.

8. Buzzer will ring when body temperature is displayed on electronic thermometer.

9. Remove plastic sheath and discard.

10. Record temperature. (Report elevated temperature to a supervisor)

11. Position client for comfort.

12. Was hands.

13. Return electronic thermometer to its storage place.

14. Report any unusual observation immediately.

*Wear gloves for measuring rectal temperatures. Follow facility policy for measuring oral temperature.

Figure 2: Average normal temperatures shown on Fahrenheit and Celsius thermometers.

Fahrenheit

_____

_____

_____

Celsius

_____

_____

_____

Fahrenheit and Celsius Comparison	
Fahrenheit	Celsius Centigrade
32	0
95	35
96	35.5
96.8	36
97.8	36.5
98.6	37
99.6	37.5
100.4	38
101.2	38.4
102.2	39
103	39.4
104	40
105	40.5
105.8	41
106.8	41.5

Rectal

The most accurate temperature reading is taken in the rectum. The normal rectal temperature is 99.6 F or 37.5 C. **Rectal** temperature is taken when patients/clients

- Are under 6 years old

- Have difficulty breathing

- Are extremely weak

- Are confused, unconscious, or senile

- Are being given oxygen

- Experience partial paralysis of the face caused by a stroke or accident

Aural

The aural temperature is also accurate, easy to use, and appropriate for the patients listed above. To measure an aural temperature, a probe is positioned in the aural canal of the ear. A normal aural temperature is 98.6 degrees F or 37 degrees C.

Axillary

The least accurate temperature is taken in the armpit. The normal temperature for this site is 97.6 degrees F or 36.4 degrees C. Use this **axillary** technique only when the temperature cannot be taken orally, aurally, or rectally. Always report a temperature that is above normal to your supervisor.

There are two types of glass thermometers. The rectal thermometer has a rounded bulb that helps prevent perforation of tissue.

Figure 3: Oral thermometer

_____

_____

_____

Figure 4: Rectal thermometer

_____

_____

_____

Chemically Treated Paper or Plastic Thermometers

This type of thermometer is read by noting the color it changes to. It is disposed of after one use.

Electronic/Digital Thermometers

This thermometer has a probe that you cover with a protective, disposable shield. The temperature is measured and registered on a screen. Electronic thermometers are quick and easy to use. There are various types of electronic equipment available. Always follow the manufacturer's instructions.

How to Read a Glass Thermometer

1. Hold the thermometer at eye level. Rotate the thermometer until you can see the column of mercury.

2. Look at the lines on the scale at the upper side of the column of mercury. Each long line represents a whole degree. There are four short lines between each of the long lines. The short lines represent 2/10 (0.2) of a degree. Only even numbers are shown on a Fahrenheit clinical thermometer.

3. If the mercury ends at one of the short lines, look to see which long line is just before it. This tells you the degree of temperature. Then add 2/10 for each short line.

4. Read a Celsius thermometer the same way. Each long line represents a degree. Each short line represents 1/10 (0.1) of a degree.

You may be asked to change a temperature from **Celsius** to **Fahrenheit** or from Fahrenheit to centigrade. If you need to make these changes, use the information in Figure 5.

Figure 5

_____

_____

_____

Sites to Take Body Temperature

Oral

The simplest and most common, convenient, and comfortable site to take a temperature are the **oral** cavity, unless you use the aural thermometer. The average normal oral temperature is 98.6 degrees F or 37 degrees C. Use the oral or aural cavity whenever possible and when the patient has

- Diarrhea

- Rectal surgery

- Fecal impaction

MEASURING AN ORAL TEMPERATURE

Rationale

As a health care worker it is important to monitor the patient's physical status. One way to determine this status by measuring the patient's temperature. This procedure explains how to measure this temperature with an oral thermometer.

ALERT: FOLLOW STANDARD PRECAUTIONS

1. Wash hands.

2. Assemble equipment.

    a. Clean oral thermometer

    b. Alcohol wipes

    c. Watch with second hand

    d. Disposable thermometer cover

3. Identify patient/client.

4. Explain what you are going to do.

5. Remove thermometer from container and apply disposable cover

6. Check reading—94 degrees F or 35 degrees C.

7. Ask patient if he or she has been smoking, eating, or drinking. If yes, wait 10 minutes before taking temperature.

8. Place thermometer under tongue.

9. Instruct client to hold with closed lips.

10. Leave in mouth for 5 minutes

11. Remove from mouth.

12. Remove and discard disposable cover and wipe thermometer from stem to tip.

13. Read thermometer correctly.

14. Wash thermometer in cool water.

15. Put away thermometer.

16. Wash hands.

17. Record temperature correctly on pad.

18. Report any unusual observation immediately.

MEASURING A RECTAL TEMPERATURE

RATIONALE

As a health care worker it is important to monitor the patient's physical status. One way to determine this status is by measuring the patient's temperature. This procedure explains how to measure this temperature rectally using a rectal thermometer.

ALERT: FOLLOW STANDARD PRECAUTIONS

1. Wash hands.

2. Assemble equipment.

    a. Clean rectal thermometer

    b. Alcohol wipes

    c. Watch with second hand

    d. Lubricant

    e. Disposable non-sterile gloves

    f. Disposable thermometer cover

3. Identify patient/client.

4. Explain what you are going to do.

5. Put on gloves.

6. Remove thermometer from container and apply disposable cover.

7. Check reading—94 degrees F or 35 degrees C.

8. Screen patient.

9. Lower backrest on bed.

10. Put lubricant on tissue and apply to bulb end of thermometer.

11. Separate buttocks.

12. Insert thermometer 1 ½ inches into rectum.

13. Hold in place 3 to 5 minutes.

14. Remove thermometer.

15. Remove and discard disposable cover and wipe thermometer from stem to tip.

16. Read thermometer correctly.

17. Wash thermometer in cool water.

18. Put away thermometer.

19. Remove and discard gloves.

20. Wash hands.

21. Record temperature correctly on pad.

22. Report any unusual observation immediately.

PALPATING A BLOOD PRESSURE

RATIONALE

As a health care worker it is important to monitor the patient's physical status. One way to determine this status is by measuring the patient's blood pressure. This procedure explains how to palpate a blood pressure so you will know how high to inflate the blood pressure cuff.

1. Wash hands.

2. Tell patient/client what you are going to do.

3. Support patient's arm palm side up on a firm surface.

4. Roll up patient's sleeve above elbow, being careful that it is not too tight.

5. Wrap wide part of cuff around client's arm directly over brachial artery. Lower edge of cuff should be 1 or 2 inches above bend of elbow.

6. Find radial pulse with your fingertips.

7. Inflate cuff until you can no longer feel radial pulse, and continue to inflate another 30 mm of mercury.

8. Open valve and slowly deflate cuff until you feel first beat of radial pulse again.

9. Observe mercury or dial reading. This is the palpatory systolic pressure. It is recorded, for example, as B/P 130 (P).

10. Deflate cuff rapidly and squeeze out all the air.

11. Using your first and second fingers, locate brachial artery. You will feel it pulsating. Place bell or diaphragm of stethoscope directly over artery. You will not hear the pulsation.

12. Tighten thumbscrew of valve to close it.

13. Hold stethoscope in place and inflate cuff until the dial points to about 20 mm above the palpated B/P.

14. Open valve counterclockwise. Let air out slowly until you hear first beat.

15. At this first sound, note reading on sphygmomanometer. This is the systolic pressure.

16. Continue to release air slowly. Note number on the indicator at which you hear last beat or the sound changes to a dull beat. This is the diastolic pressure.

17. Open valve and release all the air.

18. Remove cuff.

19. Record time and blood pressure.

20. Report any unusual observation immediately.

Summary

Blood pressure is the fourth vital sign. Many factors influence blood pressure, and an abnormal blood pressure may indicate a serious condition. It is important to be accurate in following the step-by-step instructions for taking a blood pressure, to record the blood pressure of your patient, and to report any abnormalities immediately. The mercury and aneroid apparatuses have a gauge. The gauge I marked with a series of long and short lines. The long lines are at 10-mm (millimeter) intervals. The short lines are between the long lines. These lines indicate 2 mm (millimeters) each. When you measure a blood pressure, you must do two things at one time. You listen to the heart-beat as it pulses through the artery. You also watch the gauge in order to take a reading. The blood pressure cuff is a cloth-covered rubber bladder that fills with air as the bulb is squeezed. When the cuff is inflated around the arm, it stops the flow of blood. As the pressure is relieved, the flow returns and you hear a beat. This is the systolic pressure. As the cuff continues to deflate, you hear last a beat and then silence. The last beat you hear is the diastolic pressure.

Stethoscope

When you listen to pulse sounds, you use a stethoscope. A stethoscope picks up sound when it is placed against the body. The stethoscope has earpieces, a spring to help keep the earpieces in the ears; flexible rubber tubing that carries sound, and a bell or diaphragm that magnifies sound.

PALPATING BLOOD PRESSURE

You may be asked to take a blood pressure by first palpating (feeling) the radial pulse. This allows you to determine the correct inflation pressure when inflating the cuff.

MEASURING BLOOD PRESSURE

RATIONALE

As a health care worker it is important to monitor the patient's physical status. One way to determine this status is by measuring the patient's blood pressure. This procedure explains how to determine the patient's systolic (the highest pressure) and diastolic (the lowest pressure) blood pressure.

1. Wash hands.

2. Assemble equipment.

    a. Alcohol wipes

    b. Sphygmomanometer

    c. Stethoscope

    d. Pad and pencil

3. Identify patient/client.

4. Explain what you are going to do.

5. Support patient's arm on firm surface.

6. Apply cuff correctly. (Refer to steps 4 and 5 in procedure "Palpating a Blood Pressure" on page 243.)

7. Clean earpieces on stethoscope.

8. Place earpieces in ears.

9. Locate brachial artery.

10. Tighten thumbscrew on valve.

11. Hold stethoscope in place.

12. Inflate cuff to 170 mm.

13. Open valve; if systolic sound is heard immediately, reinflate cuff to 30 mm mercury above systolic sound.

14. Note systolic at first beat.

15. Note diastolic.

16. Open valve and release air.

17. Record time and blood pressure reading correctly on pad.

18. Wash hands.

19. Wash earpieces on stethoscope.

20. Put away equipment.

21. Record blood pressure in chart.

22. Report any unusual observation immediately.

RECORDING VITAL SIGNS

Always write the temperature, pulse, and respiration in the same order:

T	P	R
98.6	**72**	**16**

Since all health care workers write vital signs in the same way, you do not need to put TPR above the figures. Write 98.6/72/16 for an oral temperature. Put an ® next to a rectal temperature (e.g., 99.6 ®) and an AX next to an axillary temperature (e.g., 97.6AX). Some facilities may have a policy and procedure requiring a T next to the aural temperature (e.g., 9836T). These symbols tell other health care workers where you measured the temperature and ensure accuracy. Always report abnormal or unusual vital signs to your supervisor.

Taking vital signs may seem routine, but the information is important to the well-being of the patient. Careful recording of vital signs is essential for the protection of the patient.

Summary

You have learned that vital signs are important indicators of the body's condition. Three of these vital signs are temperature, pulse, and respiration. There are many factors that influence TPR in the body, and it is important to be aware of them. You have learned the steps for taking temperature, pulse, and respiration, and you know how to recognize a normal TPR and an abnormal TPR. You may also be responsible for accurate measurement of O_2 in the blood. This information is essential in giving good client care and in recognizing problems with your personal health.

Blood Pressure

UNIT RATIONALE

You have learned that temperature, pulse, and respiration are signs that indicate whether or not the body is functioning within normal limits. Blood pressure is the fourth vital sign. Measuring the patient's blood pressure gives you a complete picture of his or her vital signs. A complete record of all vital signs helps in the diagnosis and treatment of the patient.

UNIT OBJECTIVES

When you have completed this unit, you will be able to do the following:

- Match vocabulary words with their correct meanings.

- Define blood pressure.

- Match descriptions of systolic and diastolic blood pressure.

- List four factors that increase blood pressure.

- List four factors that can reduce blood pressure.

- State the normal range of blood pressure.

- Demonstrate how to measure and record a blood pressure accurately.

- Explain how vital signs provide information about the patient's health.

Blood Pressure

Blood pressure is the force of the blood pushing against the walls of the blood vessels. They systolic pressure is the greatest force exerted on the walls of the arteries by the heart. This pressure is exerted when the heart is contracting. You hear the first beat when contraction occurs. The diastolic pressure is the least force exerted on the walls of the arteries by the heart. This pressure occurs as the heart relaxes between contractions. When the heart relaxes, there is no sound (beat). Blood pressure depends on the volume of blood in the circulating system, the force of the heartbeat and the condition of the arteries. When arteries lose their elasticity, they give more resistance, and the blood pressure increases. Below shows the factors that affect blood pressure.

Factors That Affect Blood Pressure

Increase Blood Pressure	Decrease Blood Pressure
Loss of elasticity in the arteries	Hemorrhage
Exercise	Inactivity
Eating	Fasting
Stimulants (e.g., medication, coffee)	Suppressants (e.g., medications that cause blood pressure to lower
Anxiety	Depression

Normal Blood Pressure

The normal blood pressure range is between 90 and 140 millimeters (mm) mercury for the systolic pressure. For the diastolic pressure, it is between 60 and 90 millimeters (mm) of mercury. When you record a blood pressure, it is written

120/80 = 120 systolic
80 diastolic

When the blood pressure is above the normal range, it is called hypertension, or high blood pressure. Hypertension is called the silent killer. It is a disease that is asymptomatic in most cases. This condition is discovered only when the patient/client has his blood pressure measured. Heredity plays a major role in patients who develop hypertension. Some of the effects are stroke, kidney problems, changes in the retina, and the heart disease. When the blood pressure is below the normal range, it is called hypotension.

Blood Pressure Apparatus

Blood pressure is measured with an instrument called a sphygmomanometer. In the word sphygmomanometer.

- Sphygmo: refers to pulse

- Mano: refers to pressure

- Meter: refers to measure

Most health care workers refer to the sphygmomanometer as a BP cuff or blood pressure cuff. There are different kinds of blood pressure apparatus:

- Mercury (This type is not seen often. In many places it is obsolete.)

- Aneroid

- Electronic/digital

Mercury Sphygmomanometer

MEASURING AN AXILLARY TEMPERATURE

RATIONALE

As a health care worker it is important to monitor the patient's physical status. One way to determine this status is by measuring the patient's temperature. This procedure explains how to measure this temperature at the axilla (under the arm).

ALERT: FOLLOW STANDARD PRECAUTIONS.

1. Wash hands.

2. Assemble equipment.

    a. Clean thermometer

    b. Alcohol wipes

    c. Watch with second hand

    d. Disposable thermometer cover

3. Identify patient/client.

4. Explain what you are going to do.

5. Remove thermometer from container and apply disposable cover.

6. Check reading—94 degrees F or 35 degrees C.

7. Place thermometer in axilla.

8. Leave in place for 10 minutes.

9. Remove thermometer.

10. Remove and discard disposable cover and wipe thermometer from stem to tip.

11. Read thermometer correctly.

12. Wash thermometer in cool water.

13. Put away thermometer.

14. Wash hands.

15. Record temperature correctly on pad.

16. Report any unusual observation immediately.

PULSE

The pulse rate indicates the number of times the heart beats in 1 minute. It is an important vital sign because it indicates how well the blood is circulating through the body. When you feel the pulse, you are feeling the pressure of the blood against the wall of the artery as the heart contracts and relaxes

Location of Pulse Points

When you count the pulse, place your fingers over an artery and squeeze gently against the bone. The pulse rate should be the same at all pulse sites.

Pulse Characteristics

Just counting the beats is not enough. You must also note the

- **Rate.** Number of pulse beats per minute.

- **Rhythm.** Is the pulse regular? Steady? Or does it skip beats?

- **Arrhythmia.** Does the pulse have uneven intervals between pulses or heartbeats?

- **Force of the beat (volume).** Is it weak, **thready**, or **bounding?** Always report a heartbeat below 60 or over 100.

Pulse Rate

Pulse rate is generally increased with exercise, age, emotional, excitement, **hemorrhage**, or elevated temperature. Drugs can increase or decrease the heart rate. When the rate is over 100 beats per minute, it is called tachycardia. When the rate is below 60 beats per minute, it is called bradycardia. When the rate is irregular, it is called arrhythmia. When you record the pulse rate, always report to your supervisor anything that is abnormal. This includes rate, rhythm, and force.

Radial Pulse

The radial pulse is the most common site for counting the pulse rate. Always count the pulse for 1 full minute. This prevents missing any abnormalities.

Apical Pulse

You may be asked to count an apical pulse. This is the pulse counted at the apex of the heart. Count an apical pulse rate when the heart is too weak to transmit a pulse that you can feel along the arteries. Count the apical heartbeat by placing the stethoscope 2 to 3 inches to the left of the sternum, just below the nipple on the chest.

Factors That Affect Pulse Rate

Increase Pulse Rate	Decrease Pulse Rate
Exercise	High level of aerobic fitness
Illness	Depression
Anxiety	Medication
Medication	
Shock	

Normal Pulse Rates

Age	Rate
Before birth	140-150
At birth	90-160
First year of life	115-130
Childhood years	80-115
Adult	60-80

COUNTING A RADIAL PULSE

RATIONALE

As a health care worker it is important to monitor the patient's physical status. One way to determine this status is by counting the patient's pulse rate. This procedure explains how to count a radial pulse.

1. Wash hands.

2. Assemble equipment.

   a. Watch with second hand

   b. Pad and pencil

3. Identify patient/client

4. Explain what you are going to do.

5. Place fingers on radial artery-do not use thumb.

6. Count pulse rate on pad immediately.

7. Wash hands.

8. Record pulse rate on chart.

9. Report any unusual observation immediately.

COUNTING AN APICAL PULSE

RATIONALE

As a health care worker it is important to monitor the patient's physical status. One way to determine this status is by counting the patient's pulse rate. This procedure explains how to count an apical pulse.

1. Assemble equipment-stethoscope.

2. Wash hands.

3. Tell patient/client what you are going to do.

4. Uncover left side of patient's chest.

5. Locate apex of heart by placing fingertips on client's chest below left nipple at about the fifth intercostal space.

6. Place stethoscope over apical region and listen for heart sounds.

7. Count the beats for 1 minute; note rate, rhythm, and strength of beat.

8. Record pulse rate on pad.

9. Wash hands.

10. Record apical pulse rate on chart.

11. Report any unusual observation immediately.

PULSE OXIMETRY

The pulse oximeter is an electronic device that determines oxygen (O_2) concentration in the hemoglobin of the arterial blood. When the O_2 concentration in the hemoglobin falls below 90%, the tissues do not have enough oxygen to function. Measuring with the oximeter allows monitoring of cardiac and respiratory patients whose blood O_2 content is an important indicator of their condition. The oximeter has light beams that pass through the tissues. The O_2 content and pulse rate are read and displayed on a monitor. Low concentrations of O_2 or a slow or rapid pulse rate cause an alarm to sound. The sensor is attached to a finger or earlobe, the forehead, the nose, or a toe. The sensor is sensitive to movement, light, and dark nail polish. Do not place a sensor over a break in the skin, a swollen area, or an area where the circulation is poor. To chart the O_2 measurement correctly, use the abbreviation SpO_2. This indicates saturation (S), pulse (p), and oxygen (O_2).

COUNTING RESPIRATIONS

RATIONALE

As a health care worker it is important to monitor the patient's physical status. One way to determine this status is by counting the patient's respiratory rate. This procedure explains how to count the number of times a patient breathes in a minute.

1. Wash hands.

2. Assemble equipment.

    a. Watch with second hand

    b. Pad and pencil

3. Identify patient/client

4. Do not explain what you are going to do.

5. Relax fingers on pulse point.

6. Observe rise and fall of chest.

7. Count respirations for 1 minute.

8. Note regularity and depth.

9. Wash hands.

10. Record respiratory rate accurately.

11. Report any unusual observation immediately.

RESPIRATION

Respiration is the process of taking oxygen (O_2) into the body and expelling carbon dioxide (CO_2) from the body. One inspiration (breathing in) and one expiration (breathing out) are considered as one respiration. When you count a patient's respiration, you do not want the patient to be aware of what you are doing. If the patient realizes that you are counting respirations, he may not breathe normally. Count the pulse rate and respirations while you are taking the temperature. When you finish counting the pulse, count the respiration rate.

Respiratory Characteristics

Age influences respiration. The rate of newborns may be 40 respirations per minute. The normal adult rate is 14 to 18 respirations per minute. Always not the following:

- **Rate**. What is the number of respirations per minute?

- **Rhythm**. Are the respirations regular or irregular?

Factors that Affect Respiration

Increase Respiration	Decrease Respiration
Exercise	Relaxation
Anxiety	Depression
Respiratory disease	Head Injury
Medication	Medication
Pain	
Heart disease (e.g., congestive heart failure)	

CHAPTER 7

UNDERSTANDING DRUG LABELS

Chapter 7

Understanding Drug Labels

Objectives

Upon mastery, you will be able to read and interpret the drug labels of the medicines you have available. To accomplish this you will also be able to:

- Find and differentiate the brand and generic names of drugs.

- Determine the dosage strength or amount of drugs by weight.

- Determine the form in which the drug is supplied.

- Identify the total volume of the drug container.

- Differentiate the total volume of the container from the dosage strength.

- Find the directions for mixing or preparing the supply strength of drugs as needed.

- Recognize the name of the drug manufacturer.

The drug order prescribes how much of a drug the patient is to receive. The nurse must prepare the order from the drugs on hand. The drug label tells how the available drug is supplied.

Look at the following common drug labels and learn to recognize pertinent information about the drugs supplied.

Brand and generic names of the drug: By law the generic name must be identified on all drug labels. Frequently the brand name is followed by the sign ® meaning the name is registered. Occasionally, only the generic name appears.

Generic Name

_____

_____

_____

Brand Name

_____

_____

_____

Dosage strength: weight of the drug

_____

_____

_____

Form: tablets, capsules, milliliters

_____

_____

_____

Supply dosage: dosage strength and form read together

_____

_____

_____

Total volume of liquid containers

_____

_____

_____

Directions for mixing or reconstituting powdered forms of drugs.

_____

_____

_____

Oral Dosage of Drugs

Objectives

Upon mastery, you will be able to calculate the oral dosages of drugs. To accomplish this you will also be to:

- Convert all units of measurement to the same system and same size units.

- Consider what is the reasonable amount of the drug to be administered.

- Use the formula $\underline{d} \times Q$ to calculate drug dosage.
  $\quad\quad\quad\quad h$

- Allow for no more than 10 percent variance in determined dosages when using approximate equivalents.

- Calculate the number of tablets or capsules that are contained in prescribed dosages.

- Calculate the volume of liquid per dose when the prescribed dosage is in solution form.

Tablets and Capsules

Drugs prepared in tablet and capsule form come in the strengths or dosages in which they are commonly given. It is desirable to obtain the drug in the strength of the dosage ordered, or in multiples of that dosage. When necessary, scored tablets (those marked for division) can be divided in halves or quarters.

When a choice is possible, the strength of the drug should be selected so that the fewest number of tablets or capsules can be administered.

Example: The doctor's order reads: Ilosone(erythromycin estolate) 250 mg p.o. q.i.d

Ilosone chewable tablets come in strengths of 125 milligrams per tablet and 250 milligrams per tablet. When both strengths are available, the nurse should select the 250 milligram strength and give one tablet for each dose.

RULE:

To compute the correct dosage of the drug ordered, use the following three simple steps.

Step 1. Be sure that all measures are in the same system, and all units are in the same size, converting when necessary.

MEDICINE FOR THE MIND: INTRODUCTION TO HEALTH CAREERS (WORKBOOK)

Step 2. Carefully consider what is the reasonable amount of the drug that should be administered.

Step 3. Calculate the drug dosage using the formula <u>D</u> (desired) X Q (quantity) = X (amount to be administered). H (have)

Look at each of the three steps separately

Step 1. Be sure that all measures are in the same system, and all units are in the same size converting when necessary.

Step 1 means that medication orders written and supplied in the same system but in different size units will need to be converted to the same size. For instance, a drug ordered in grams but supplied in milligrams will need to be converted to the same size unit. In most cases, it is more practical to change to the smaller unit (g to mg) since this usually eliminates the decimal or fraction and keeps the calculation in whole numbers.

For example, 0.5vg = 500mg (Equivalent: 1 g = 1000 mg).

_____

_____

_____

If the medication order is written in the apothecaries' system and the medication is supplied in the metric system, you must recall the approximate equivalents and convert both amounts to the same system.

The rule of thumb is to convert to the system of measure for the supply dosage you have available on hand. You will find that you will, in fact, convert apothecaries' or house-hold systems to the metric system. This is true since the metric system is the predominant system of measure for drug preparations.

For example, the physician may order phenobarbital gr ¼ p.o. and the drug you have available on hand is labeled phenobarbital 15 mg per tablet. To determine how many tablets to give the patient, you must first convert gr ¼ to the metric equivalent.

Gr ¼ =15 mg (equivalent gr I = 60 mg)

Step 2. Carefully consider what is a reasonable amount of the drug that should be administered.

Once you have converted all units to the same system and size, step 2 asks you to logically conclude what amount should be given. Before you go on to step 3, you should be able to picture in your mind the exact amount of medication to be administered. At least, you should be able to make a very close approximation, such as more or less than one table (capsule, milliliter, dram). Basically, step 2 says. "think"

In the preceding example, once you have completed the conversions, you can readily reason for the correct amount of tablets to administer. You would give one table of phenobarbital.

Step 3. Calculate the drug using the formula D (desired) X Q (quantity) = X (amount to be administered) H (have)

Always double-check your "reasonable" answer with the simple formula given in step 3. D (desired) X Q = X. In this formula, D represents the dose desired or the dose

H (have)

Ordered. H represents the dosage strength of the drug you have on hand in the drug container.

Q represents the quantity (capacity or volume) of the dosage on hand. In solving dosage problems when the drug on hand is supplied in tablets, capsules, or caplets, the volume of the dosage on hand is always "I." The supply dosage or dosage you have on hand is per one capsule or tablet. Thus, if a drug prescription is for a 500 milligram dose Amoxil and you have amoxicillin (Amoxil) on hand in 250 milligram capsules, this means that there are 250 milligrams in each capsule. Use the formula to determine how many capsules should be administered.

Dose Desired or ordered X Quantity of dose you have on hand = AMOUNT to

Dose you HAVE on hand

Administer or, more simply

$$\frac{D \text{ (Desired)}}{H \text{ (Have)}} \times Q \text{ (Quantity)} = X \text{ (Amount to Give)}$$

$$\text{Or } \frac{500 \text{ mg}}{250 \text{ mg}} \times 1 \text{ capsule} = \frac{500}{250} = \text{Give 2 capsules}$$

RULE:

The formula method for dosage calculations is:

$$\frac{D}{H} \times Q = X$$

Steps 1, 2, and 3 can be used to solve all oral or parenteral dosage calculation problems encountered. It is important that you develop the ability to reason for the answer logically as well as learn to use the $\frac{D}{H} \times Q$ formula.

Errors are often made unknowingly because nurses rely solely on a formula rather than asking themselves first what the answer should be. As a nurse you are expected to be able to reason sensible, problem-solve, and justify your judgments rationally. Use the formula as a tool to validate the dosage you anticipate should be given. If your reasoning is sound, you will find the dosages you compute make sense and are accurate.

INTERROGATIVES	PALABRAS INTERROGATIVAS
1. How?	Como?
2. How far?	A que distancia?
3. How often?	Con que frecuencia?
4. How much?	Cuanto?
5. How many?	Cuantos?
6. How long?	Cuanto tiempo?
7. How many times?	Cuantas veces?
8. What?	Que?
9. What else?	Que mas?
10. What for?	Para que?
11. When?	Cuando?
12. Where?	Donde?
13. From where?	De donde?
14. To where?	Adonde?
15. Which?	Cual?
16. Which (ones)?	Cuales?
17. Who?	Quien?
18. To Whom?	A quien?
19. Whose?	De quien?
20. Why?	Por que?

TITLES	TITULOS
Mr.	Senor
Mrs.	Senora
Miss	Senorita
Family Member (Relative)	Miembros de la Familia (Parientes)
Grandfather	abuelo
Grandmother	abuela
Mother	la madre, la mama
Father	el padre, el papa
Parents	los padres
Son	el hijo
Daughter	la hija
Children	los hijos, los nino
Sister	la hermana
Brother	el hermano
Cousin	el (la) primo(a)
Father in law	el suegro
Mother in law	la suegra
In laws	los suegros
Brother in law	el cunado
Sister in law	la cunada
Niece	la sobrina
Nephew	el sobrino
Husband	el esposo, el marido, "el Viejo"(slang)
Wife	la esposa, la mujer "la vieja" (slang)
Aunt	la tia
Uncle	el tio
Daughter in law	la nuera
Son in law	el yerno

Medical Personnel — **Personal Medico**

Doctor	el doctor, el medico la doctora, la medica
Nurse	el enfermero, la enfermera
Therapist	el terapista, la terapista
Paramedic	el paramédico, la paramedico

Orderly	el ayudante, la ayudante
Hospital	volunteer el voluntario, la voluntaria

Greetings and social amenties **Saludos**

Good morning	Buenos días
Good afternoon	Buenas tardes
Good evening	Buenas tardes, Buenas noches
Good night	Buenas noches
Goodbye	Adios
Hello	Hola
Let me introduce myself	Permitame presentarme
My name Is	Me llamo
I am	Soy
What is your name?	Como se llama usted?
Pleased to meet you	Mucho gusto
Likewise	Igualmente
How are you?	Como esta usted?
How do you feel?	Como se siente usted?
So, so	Asi, asi (Regular)
Better than yesterday	Mejor que ayer
Please	Por favor
Thank you	Gracias
You're welcome	De nada (por nada)
My deepest sympathy	Mi sentido pésame
I am sorry	Lo siento
What a pity	Que lastima!
Congratulations	Feliciadades!
Do you speak English?	Habla usted ingles?
Please speak more slowly.	Hable mas despacio, por favor
What's the matter?	Que le pasa?
Do you want something?	Desea usted algo?
Come in	Pase usted (Entre usted)
Sit down	Tome asiento
What can I do for you?	En que le puedo ayudar?

COMPLETIONS

Anything, something	algo
Bad, badly	mal, muy mal
Before	ante
Better	mejor
Earlier	mas temprano
Enough	bastante, suficient
Everyday	todos los dias, cada dia
Fast	rapido
Fever	fiebre, calentura
Here	aqui, aca
It (not expressed as a subject)	lo
Last night	anoche
Late	tarde
Later	mas tarde
A little	un poco, un poquito
Less	menos
A lot	mucho
More	mas
Never, ever	nunca, jamas, alguna vez
Now	ahora
Slow	despacio
Soon	pronto
That	eso
Sample, specimen	muestra
There	alla
This	esto
This morning	esta manana
This afternoon	esta tarde
Tonight	esta noche
Today	hoy
tonight	esta noche

Medical Terminology Glossary

Accurate: exact, correct, or pecise.

Afebrile: temperature is within normal range

Anesthesia: loss of feeling or sensation.

Antiseptic: substance that slows or stops the growth of microorganisms.

Apex: pointed end of something (e.g. the pointed end of the heart is called the apex of the heart).

Apnea: not breathing

Apparatus: equipment needed to perform a task (e.g. blood pressure apparatus includes a blood pressure cuff and a stethoscope).

Asepsis: sterile condition, free from all germs.

Asymptomatic: without visible symptoms

Axillary: referring to the armpit.

Blood pressure: highest and lowest pressure against the walls of blood vessels.

Bounding: leaping, strong, or forceful (e.g. a very strong pulse is a bounding pulse).

Calibration: standard measure (e.g. each line on a thermometer or a ruler is a calibration).

Celsius: measure of heat; in medicine a Celsius thermometer is sometimes used to measure body heat. Also called centigrade.

Convents: establishments of nuns

Custodial: marked by watching and protecting rather than seeking to cure.

Diastolic pressure: lowest pressure against the blood vessels of the body. It is measured between contractions.

Dissection: act or process of dividing, taking apart

Excretion: process of eliminating waste material.

Exorcise: to force out evil spirits.

Facilities: places designed or built to serve a special function (e.g. hospital, clinic, doctor's office)

Fahrenheit: measure of heat; in medicine a Fahrenheit thermometer is often used to measure body heat.

Febrile: temperature is elevated

Gauge: standard scale for measurement

Geriatric: pertaining to old age.

Hemorrhage: large amount of bleeding

Hypotension: low blood pressure

Hypothermia: temperature is below normal

Inflated: to swell or fill up with air

Intravenously: directly into a vein.

Microorganisms: organisms so small that they can only be seen through a microscope.

Millimeters: measure of length

Monasteries: homes for men following religious standards.

Noninvasive: not involving penetration of the skin.

Observation: act of watching

Obsolete: out of date

Oral: referring to the mouth.

Oxidation: the mixing together of oxygen and another element.

Predators: organisms or beings that destroy.

Pyrexia: above-normal temperature

Pyrogenic: any substance that produces fever

Quackery: practice of pretending to cure diseases.

Recipient: one who receives.

Rectal: referring to the far end of the large intestine just above the anus.

Stethoscope: Instrument used to hear sound in the body (e.g. heartbeat, lung sounds, bowel sounds).

Superstitious: trusting in magic or chance.

Sphygmomanometer: measuring device used to measure the pressure against the arteries of the body.

Systolic pressure: highest pressure against blood vessels. Represented by first heart sound or beat heard when taking a blood pressure

Tachypnea: abnormally fast respirations

Thread: weak, barely-felt pulse; thin, like a thread

TPR: stands for "temperature, pulse, respiration."

CHAPTER 8

EMPLOYABILITY & LEADERSHIP

Chapter 8

Employability and Leadership

Unit 1

Job-Seeking Skills

UNIT RATIONALE

Before you apply the skills you have learned, you must find a job and be hired as an employee. It is important to learn the skills needed to find a job and to keep a job. This enables you to practice the health care career that you worked so hard to learn.

UNIT OBJECTIVES

When you have completed this unit, you will be able to do the following:

- List seven places to seek employment opportunities and explain the benefits of each.

- Explain four ways to contact an employer.

- Name three occasions when a cover letter is used.

- List eight items required on a resume.

- Identify seven items generally requested on a job application form.

- Write a cover letter and a resume.

- Complete a job application.

- List five do's and five don'ts of job interviewing.

FINDING A JOB

Looking for and finding a job takes planning and requires the use of many skills. In this chapter, you learn the steps to follow when you are ready to find a job. These skills give you the tools to be successful in job seeking and save you a lot of time.

YOUR VOCATIONAL PORTFOLIO

As time approaches to begin your search for a job, review your portfolio notebook. Obtain a new cover and section dividers so your finished portfolio has a clean, crisp look. Identify the items that best reflect your knowledge level, skills, and personality. When you complete your resume and other portfolio requirements place them in the appropriate section of your new portfolio.

PLACES TO SEEK EMPLOYMENT

Newspaper ads. Jobs in health care careers appear in newspaper ads. When you look for a job in the newspaper, turn to the classified ads and look under "Help Wanted." There are different ways of listing jobs. Some papers list all health care positions under "Medical." Others list them under a particular job. You also need to become familiar with some of the abbreviations used by newspapers.

Common Abbreviations	
Appl.	applicant
Asst.	assistant
Cert.	certified
Exp.	Experience
FT	full time
Immed.	Immediately
Incl.	included
Lic.	Licensed
N.A.	nurse aide
PT	part time

Directly to the employer

If you are looking for a position in a laboratory, you might apply directly to a medical laboratory. If you want to work in a hospital, you go to the **personnel** department. The Yellow Pages of your phone book offer an excellent resource of possible employers.

Friends and relatives

You may know of someone working in the health care field who can suggest a place to apply or who can introduce you to a possible employer.

School counselors

Many schools have career counselors and/or work experience counselors. They are a good resource for the types of jobs available in your community.

School bulletin boards

If you have a career center or a bulletin board where jobs are listed, be sure to check it daily.

Employment agencies

There are both public and private employment agencies. Employers call these agencies to list the job openings that they have. A public agency does not charge a fee; however, a private agency charges either the employer or the person seeking a position. The Yellow Pages list employment agencies, and some of them specialize in health care careers. The public agencies are listed in the white pages under "Government Agencies."

Internet

If you have access to a computer that is connected to the Internet, go to Search and type in the words "job search" or "job link."

WAYS TO CONTACT AN EMPLOYER

Now that you know where to look for a job, you need to know how to make the contact and how to present yourself.

Telephone

If you have a lead on a possible job, you may choose to call for an appointment. Give your name and the job you are interested in and ask when you may come in to apply.

Cover Letter

You may be asked to send a letter in order to apply for a particular position. You need a cover letter when

- You are applying for a job that is out of town.

- You are answering a newspaper advertisement.

- A potential employer requests a letter.

   Your cover letter is a sales letter. You want to sell yourself to the employer in order to get an interview. (A sample cover letter is shown in Table 1.1.) Your letter should

- Be neat

- Have all the words spelled correctly

- State where you heard about the job opening

- State wheat you are applying fro and why you are qualified for this specific position

- Give a brief overview of your education, experience, and qualifications

- Refer to your portfolio with work samples, skills check off lists, and evaluations

- Request an interview

- Give your address and phone number

Resume

In addition to your cover letter, it is helpful for a potential employer to have more details about you and your qualifications. This is accomplished by preparing a resume (See the example in Table 1.2.) A resume includes the following:

- Your name, address, phone number, and message number

- Career plans

- Details about your education

- Your past work experience-paid or unpaid

- What honors you have earned

- What activities you like

- Skills, strengths, and abilities

- References (always ask permission to use someone as a reference)

Job Application

Most employers require that you fill out an application. When you fill out a job application, you give the employer needed information and also have an opportunity to demonstrate that you are neat and well organized. Use the information in your vocational portfolio to fill out an application. Included should be

- Your complete address with the zip code.

- Your Social Security number.

- Your phone number or a number where you can be reached.

- A list of the schools you have attended, with dates.

- A list of any special training that you have.

- A prepared list of any past jobs, the address of the employer, the dates you worked there, and what your duties were.

- A list of people who can give you a reference. Be certain that you have their addresses and phone numbers. Also be certain that you have asked permission to use them as a reference.

There are also other ways that you can prepare. Be sure that you

- Carry a pen—do not use a pencil.

- Read the application all the way through.

- Print unless you are told to write.

- Spell accurately.

- Answer every question. Put "NA" (not applicable) in the space to show that you did not overlook the question.

- Recheck for errors.

INTERVIEW

The interviewer wants to be sure that you are the best fit for the job. She is assessing your skills from the time she receives your resume. Her focus during the interview is to determine if your explanations and behaviors match the job requirements. This evaluation occurs throughout the interview process, even when conversation is about the weather or hobbies. It is important to make a good first impression. The following guidelines tell you what to do and what not to do during an interview.

Interview Guidelines

Follow these guidelines for a positive interview experience.

- Be well groomed.

- Dress neatly and appropriately (no jeans).

- Be on time.

- Greet the interviewer by name, and smile.

- Shake hands firmly.

- Stand until asked to sit.

- Answer questions truthfully and sincerely.

- Be enthusiastic.

- Do not chew gum.

- Do not criticize former employers or teachers.

- Look at the interviewer when you talk.

- Do not talk about personal problems.

- When the interview is over, thank the interviewer and leave quickly.

Interview Preparation

The interviewer expects you to answer a variety of questions pertinent to the job you are applying for. Be prepared to give at least three examples of your behavior in various situations. Each experience should describe the

- **Situation.** What exactly happened?

- **Behavior.** What did you do?

- **Outcome.** What were the results?

Read the following questions and determine how to answer them.

- Tell me about the most difficult decision you made at school or work in the last few months.

- Tell me how you get along with people at school or work.

- Tell me about the most difficult job or school task you've done. Why was it difficult? How did you get past the difficulties?

- Explain a recent situation that demonstrates your ability to be a team player.

- Describe a situation in which you had to work under pressure. What kind of pressure were you facing? How did you handle the situation? What was the outcome?

- Describe a situation where you had to be very flexible.

After the Interview

The interviewer will do a reference check to verify that your resume and application are honest and accurate. She will also rate your responses to help her make a decision about which candidate is best for the job. The following is an example of interview rating scale with topics.

	Excellent	Average	Not Acceptable
Appearance			
Manner			
Qualifications			
Experience			

Job fit

After the interview, send a letter of thanks to the interviewer. (See the example Table 1.3.) This lets the interviewer know that you are interested in position and it may increase your chance of getting the job.

Finding a job and then getting a job take effort on your part. Careful planning is the key to your success, and you will be glad that you took time to prepare yourself.

SUMMARY

Finding a job requires effort on your part. When you decide to look for a job, check the newspaper; go to a personnel department; ask friends, relatives, and your school counselor if they know of an opening; check employment agencies and bulletin boards; and search the Internet. After finding a possible opening, contact the employer. Call for an appointment, or send a cover letter with your resume. You will also have to fill out a job application.

The last step is your interview with the employer. There are some important rules to follow when you go to an interview. After your interview, send a thank-you not to the interviewer.

UNIT 2

KEEPING A JOB

Unit Rationale

You spend a lot of time and effort learning the skills for a career in health care. You also spend a lot of time and effort finding a job and then getting the job. Now that you have the job, you want to keep it. Employers have very specific things that they are looking for in an employee. The information in this unit tells what these things are and how you can be a good employee.

Unit Objectives

When you have completed this unit, you will be able to do the following:

- Define vocabulary words.

- List four employer responsibilities.

- List four responsibilities of a good employee.

Summary

Once you acquire a job, you and your employer agree to work together to accomplish the job you are hired to do. Your behavior reflects your attitude and values. Continually evaluate your actions using the Dignity, Excellence, Service, and Fairness/Justice criteria as a measure of your progress in the work environment. Be a team player by respecting your co-workers and encouraging them to do the best job they can do.

Unit 3

BECOMING A PROFESSIONAL LEADER

UNIT RATIONALE

Student and professional health care organizations enhance the delivery of compassionate, high-quality care by providing knowledge, skill, and leadership development. Committed students and professionals seek opportunities provided by these organizations to keep current and to provide patients with good-quality care.

UNIT OBJECTIVES

When you have completed this chapter, you will be able to do the following:

- Define vocabulary words.

- Name the three main benefits of being a member of a student health vocational organization.

- Name six benefits of being a member of a professional organization.

- Identify ways to find a professional organization.

- Identify steps to becoming a leader.

- Define HOSA and SkillsUSA

- Summarize why you plan to participate in a student and professional organization.

MEMBERSHIP IN AN ORGANIZATION

Membership in your student or professional organization gives you an opportunity to gain occupational knowledge and skills. It also provides opportunities to develop leadership skills. Some of the skills that you learn include the following:

- Professional ethics

- Communication and interpersonal relations

- Leadership skills

- Ability to recognize and initiate change

- How to organize activities and people

- Time management

- Establishing priorities

- Budgeting

- Fund raising

- Current health issues

Health Occupations Students of America (HOSA)

Health Occupations Students of America (HOSA) is the student organization for health occupation students at the secondary, postsecondary, adult, and college level. Among HOSA's primary goals are to

- Promote career opportunities in the health care industry

- Enhance and promote the delivery of quality health care to all people

- Encourage all health occupations students and instructors to be actively involved in current health care issues

Skills Competitions

HOSA provides many opportunities for students to learn and achieve. One such opportunity is the skills competitions. Competitions are at three levels-local, state, and national-with students advancing on to the next levels by winning the previous ones. HOSA offers 44 different events divided into categories based on the curriculum. Competitive event categories include:

- Category I: Health occupations related to

    a. Medical math

    b. Medical spelling

    c. Medical terminology

    d. Dental spelling

    e. Dental terminology

- Category II: Health occupations skills such as

    a. Medical assisting-clerical

    b. Medical assisting-clinical

    c. Dental assisting

    d. Nursing assisting

    e. Practical/vocational nursing

    f. CPR/first aid

- Category III: Individual leadership skills including

    a. Extemporaneous speaking

    b. Extemporaneous health display

    c. Extemporaneous writing

    d. Job-seeking skills

    e. Prepared speaking

- Category IV: Team leadership demonstrated by

    a. Community awareness

    b. HOSA Bowl participation

- Category V: Recognition

    a. Outstanding HOSA chapter

    b. National recognition program

Competition requirements include the following:

- Student must be an active HOSA member.

- Student must be identified as either a secondary student (currently enrolled in a high school) or a postsecondary student (graduate from high school or over 18 years of age).

    Students attending HOSA functions follow a strict code of conduct and official HOSA uniform and competitive event dress codes. Experiencing the challenges, structure, and competition in HOSA teaches students how to reach for and achieve their highest potential.

Vocational Industrial Clubs of America (VICA)

Skills USA-Vica is a national organization serving more than 250,000 high school and college students and professional members who are enrolled in training programs in technical, skilled, and service occupations, including health occupations. SKillsUSA has more than a quarter million student members annually, organized into 13,000 chapters and 54 state and territorial associations (including the District of Columbia, Puerto Rico, Guam and the Virgin Islands.). For additional information see the Website at www.skillsUSA.org.

Purpose Statement

SkillsUSA prepares America's high performance workers. It provides quality educational experiences for students in leadership, teamwork, citizenship and character development. It builds and reinforces self-confidence, work attitudes and communications skills. It emphasizes total quality at work, high ethical standards, superior work skills. It emphasizes total quality at work, high ethical standards, superior work skills, life-long education and pride in the dignity of work. SkillsUSA also promotes understanding of the free enterprise system and involvement in community service activities.

Programs

SkillsUSA programs include local, state, and national competitions in which students demonstrate occupational and leadership skills. During the annual national level SkillsUSA Championships, more than 4,100 students compete in 73 occupational and leadership skill areas. SKillsUSA programs also help to establish industry standards for job skill training in the classroom.

The Total Quality Curriculum enhances SkillsUSA's Quality at Work movement by preparing students for the world of work starting in the classroom. The curriculum emphasizes the competencies and essential workplace basic skills identified by employers and the U.S. Secretary of Labor's Commission on Achieving Necessary Skills(SCANS). The Professional Development Program is a self-paced curriculum for secondary and college students. It teaches skills such as effective communication and management, teamwork, networking, workplace ethics, job interviewing and more. The curriculum involves local industry and academics and can be used in day-trades, apprenticeship training, cooperative education, school-to-work, academic and special needs programs.

National Program of Work

The National Program of Work sets the pace for SkillsUSA-VICA nationwide. All programs are in some way related to the following seven major goals. The expectations is that each chapter will carry out this program of work.

Professional development

To prepare each SkillsUSA-VICA member for entry into the work force and provide a foundation for success in a career. Becoming a professional does not stop with acquiring a skill, but involves an increased awareness of the meaning of good citizenship and the importance of labor and management in the world of work.

Community service

To promote and improve good will and understanding among all segments of this community through services donated by SkillsUSA-VICA chapters, and to instill its members a lifetime commitment to community service.

Employment

To increase student awareness of quality job practices and attitudes, and to increase the opportunities for employer contact and eventual employment.

Ways and means

To plan and participate in fund-raising activities to allow all members to carry the chapter's projects.

SkillsUSA Championships

To offer students the opportunity to demonstrate their skills and be recognized for them through competitive activities in occupational areas and leadership.

Public relations

To make the general public aware of the good work that students in career and technical education are doing to better themselves and their community, state, nation and world.

Social activities

To increase cooperation in the school and community through activities that allows SkillsUSA-VICA members to get to know each other in something other than a business or classroom setting.

PROFESSIONAL ORGANIZATIONS

Professional organizations help professionals keep current in the latest technology and trends. Being aware of the advantages offered through involvement in such organizations motivates health care workers to become active in the professional group for their chosen occupation.

There are numerous professional organizations for the health care worker. Most organizations have a local chapter, state chapter, and national chapter. Each supports the other and all work toward common goals. Belonging to a professional organization provides the following benefits:

- Updates on new technological advances

- Communication with other geographical areas

- Shared resources

- Resources for employment opportunities

- Current legislative issues

- Interaction with other health professionals

- Pooled money to accomplish changes for the good of the occupation/profession

- Power as united group to encourage positive change

- Development of new ideas that support growth

When your classes are complete, find your professional organization by

- Referring to Chapter 2 of this book

- Asking fellow employees

- Reading the bulletin boards at work

- Reading your professional journals

- Reading brochures

- Attending occupationally related in-service programs

- Checking the Occupational Outlook Handbook

Leadership

Becoming a leader in your occupational area takes time and patience. To become a leader you must take several important steps. These include the following:

- Developing a superior skill level

- Becoming a decision maker

- Being a good communicator

- Developing a balanced focus on tasks and people

Tom Peters, author of a Passion for Excellence, says:

"**A leader is a** . . . . . . **A leader is not a** . . . .

Cheerleader	cop
Enthusiast	referee
Nurturer	devil's advocate
Coach	naysayer
Facilitator	pronouncer"

A true leader unites people and works toward positive outcomes.

SUMMARY

Participation in HOSA or SkillsUSA is an important part of your career development and professionalism. As a member, you are introduced to various health careers, develop a responsible attitude toward your community, develop knowledge and skills for the work world, and gain self-confidence.

Membership prepares you to be a leader in your chosen occupation; it also helps you prepare to become a valuable member of your professional organization when you join the workforce.

To become a leader you must develop superior skill levels, become a decision maker, be a good communicator, and develop a balanced focus on tasks and people.

For more information, write

National HOSA
6021 Morriss Road
Suite 111
Flower Mound, TX 75028
(800)321 4672
Fax (972)874-0063
Website:http://www.hosa.org
Email: info@hosa.org

SkillsUSA-VICA
P.O. Box 3000
Leesburg, VA 20177-0300
(703) 777-8810
Fax (703) 7777-8999
Website: http://www.skillsusa.org
email: anyinfo@skillsusa.org

CHAPTER 9

BECOMING A LEADER

Chapter 9

Becoming a Leader

Rationale

It is important for students to understand the benefits of membership in a student health organization. Student organizations enhance your learning by providing exciting and varied experiences.

Objectives

When you complete this chapter you will:

- Name the four main benefits of being a member of a student health vocational organization

- Name five benefits of being a member of a professional organization.

- Identify ways to find a professional organization.

MEMBERSHIP IN AN ORGANIZATION

Membership in your vocational student organization or professional organization gives you an opportunity to develop your leadership skills. These skills are useful in your personal life and in your work environment. The skills you learn include:

- Effective communication

- Ability to lead others

- Ability to recognize and initiate change

- Organize activities and people

- Time management

- Establishing priorities

- Budgeting

- Fund raising

There are many student vocational organizations available for interested students. These organizations focus their attention in a variety of vocational areas. The range spans form business to homemaking, agriculture, health, and industrial arts. In this chapter we discuss those organizations with a focus on health. The national student health organizations available to you are:

- Health Occupation Students of America (HOSA)

- Vocational Industrial Club of America (VICA), Health Occupations Component

- These organizations have established purposes and goals to meet the needs of students in health-related occupations. Some of the purposes that are common to each of the organizations are to:

- Promote high standards in ethics, skills, scholarship, and safety

- Foster respect for the dignity of work

- Provide recognition and prestige that will foster physical, mental, and social well-being

- Develop leadership abilities through various activities

- Promote involvement in current health care issues

  Student health organizations offer exceptional benefits to their members. Some of these include:

- Introduction to various health careers

- Developing a responsible attitude through service to the community

- Available guidance that develops knowledge, skills, and characteristics necessary in preparing to be a health care worker

- Help for students to gain self-confidence through the development of leadership skills

Membership in a student health organization provides students with an opportunity to travel and compete in skills competition. Competition is held at three levels:

- The first level is local competition; those who win go on to the second level.

- The second level is state competition; those who win go on the third level.

- The third level is national competition.

- Competitive events usually include:

    a. Health-occupations-related events

    b. Basic first aid and CPR

    c. Extemporaneous health display

    d. Dental and medical spelling

    e. Dental and medical terminology

- Health occupations skills events

    a. Dental assisting

    b. Medical assisting

    c. Nursing assisting

    d. Practical nursing

- Individual leadership events

    a. Extemporaneous speaking

    b. Job-seeking skills

    c. Prepared speaking

- Team leadership events

    a. Community awareness project

    b. Parliamentary procedure

Each organization has established official colors, dress codes, and emblems. The unity in dress and an official emblem promote pride and professionalism. Membership in one of these organizations helps you understand the importance of your involvement in the professional organization related to your career area. You can make a difference by being active in your professional organization after graduation.

PROFESSIONAL ORGANIZATIONS

Professional organizations assist professionals to be updated in the latest state of the art technology and trends. Being aware of the advantages offered through involvement in such organizations motivates health care workers to become active in the professional group for their chosen occupation.

There are numerous professional organizations for the health care worker. Most organizations have a local chapter, state chapter, and a national chapter. Each supports the other and all work toward common goals. Belonging to a professional organization provides the following benefits.

- Updates on new technological advances

- Communicating from other geographical areas

- Sharing resources

- Resource for employment opportunities

- Updates of new legislation

- Interaction with their health professional

- Pooled money to accomplish changes for the good of the occupation

- Power as a united group to encourage positive change

- Develop new ideas that support growth

    When you complete your classes you will want to find a professional organization. How do you find a professional organization? Some of the ways to find information on your professional organization are to:

- Ask fellow employee

- Read the bulletin boards at work

- Read your professional journals

- Take time to read brochures that come in the mail

- Attend occupationally related in-service programs

- Check the Occupation Outlook Handbook

SUMMARY

Participation in student organizations is an important part of your career development. As a member, you are introduced to various health careers, develop a responsible attitude toward your community, develop knowledge and skills for the work world, and gain self-confidence.

Membership prepares you to be a leader in your chosen occupation; it also helps you prepare to become a valuable member to your professional organization when you join the work force.

For further information, write:

- Vocational Industrial Clubs of America, Inc.

  P.O. Box 3000
  Leesburg, VA 22075
  703-777-8810

- National HOSA Office

  4108 Amon Center
  Suite 202
  Fort Worth, TX 76155
  817-354-5047

CHAPTER 10

THE SPECIAL SENSES

Chapter 10

The Special Senses
The Sources of Information

It's a Fact:

Vision is so sensitive that, on a clear moonless night, a person n a mountain can detect the striking of a match 50 miles away.

CHAPTER OVERVIEW

In this chapter we discuss the five special senses: vision, hearing, smell, taste, and touch, and their unique structures and sensation mechanisms.

THE SENSE OF VISION

The organ of vision is the eye, with its various accessory organs, such as the extrinsic muscles, the eyelids, and the tear apparatus. Strictly speaking, the eye includes on eye the bulb of the eye (the eyeball) and the optic nerve, which connects it with the brain. This system constitutes the essential part of the organ of vision. (The term optic refers to the eye, as do the combining forms oculo and ophthalmo.)

The eye is the most important sense organ in the body. It is from the eye that we receive most of our information, not only in what we can see around us or in the near distance, but also in what we learn through the printed word.

The eyeball occupies the front half of the orbital cavity, where it is embedded (cushioned) in fat and connective tissue. The eyeballs lie on either side of the root of the nose, and are almost sphere-shaped. Attached to the eyeball and contained in its orbital cavity are the optic nerve, ocular muscles, and certain other nerves and vessels. A soft mucous membrane, called the conjunctiva, covers the anterior (or exposed) third of the eyeball, and lines the eyelids. The eyes are protected by the eyelids (referred to as a palpebrae, combining form is (blepharo), which are fringed with eyelashes (referred to as cilia); above the eyes another row of hairs, usually arched in appearance, forms the eyebrows (referred to a supercilia). The eyes are moistened and kept clean by the tears from the lacrimal glands, and the eyelids blink frequently to spread the secretions of the lacrimal glands over the external surface of the eye, keeping it moist.

Movement of the eyeball is by six slender extrinsic muscles, attached to each eye, that act together. The movement of opening the eyes, however, is confined to the upper lid. The eyes are free to move in any direction, upward, downward, and sideways, or the gaze may be fixed and straight ahead.

The eyeball is like a hollow sphere whose wall is made up of three concentric coats and whose cavity is filled with transparent refracting media (tissues and fluid that transmit light). The outer fibrous coat, the sclera, has a white opaque, posterior portion and a transparent anterior portion called the cornea. The intermediate coat, the choroid, is vascular and pigmented, and divided into a posterior portion and a smaller anterior portion, which has three structures, the ciliary body, the suspensory ligament, and the iris. The retina (internal coat), is the light-sensitive layer that is made up of differentiated nervous receptors continuous with the optic nerve. Three transparent refractive media fill the optic cavity; the vitreous body (semi-gelatinous substance contained in a thin, clear membrane) between the retina and the lens, and two aqueous humor (watery fluid) chambers anterior to the lens.

The eye is like a camera, with an opening in front, the pupil, that lets light in, a crystalline lens behind the pupil focusing the rays of light to form an image on the retina, which contains the vision sense organs, the rods and cones. The optic nerve carries the impulses from the rods and cones to the visual area.

Structures of the Eye

Sclera

The sclera is the white, opaque portion of the eye, "the white of the yey," and constitutes the posterior five-sixths of the eyeball. It is composed of white fibrous tissue and fine elastic fibers, with the front portion covered by a membrane called the conjunctiva, through which small, superficial blood vessels can be seen. In children, the sclera is often very thin and allows the underlying choroidal pigment to show through, giving the sclera a bluish cast, and in the aged, one often sees a yellowish cast. The conjunctiva surfaces are lubricated and washed by the tears secreted by the lacrimal glands.

Cornea

The cornea is the anterior, transparent portion of the fibrous coat of the eyeball through which light enters the eye. It is nearly circular in shape, and its marked curvature makes it bulge with a dome-like protrusion that varies among individuals and diminishes somewhat with age. It is devoid of blood and lymph vessels, except at the extreme periphery, and this lack of vascularity makes the cornea subject to infection after injury.

Choroid

The choroid is located between the sclera and retina, and its posterior part is a thin membrane with a rich vascular layer. The cells of the choroid are filled with a melanin, a black or dark brown pigment, which gives it a dark brown appearance. Extra light is absorbed by the pigment which helps to prevent blurring of an image by internally reflected light. The chief function of the choroid is to maintain the nutrition of the retina through its capillary plexus and numerous small arteries and veins.

Ciliary Body

The ciliary body, an extension of the choroid, is a thickened portion of the vascular layer which extends from the visual layer to the iris. The ciliary body is a wedge-shaped, flattened ring, with muscles connected the suspensory ligament that attaches the lens to it, and processes (ridges) that secrete the aqueous humor (fluid). The ciliary processes consist of a rich vascular plexus embedded in pigmented stroma (connective tissue). Focusing on far or near objects (called accommodation), is accomplished through changing the shape of the lens by action of the ciliary muscles.

Suspensory Ligament

The suspensory ligament is the second structure of the anterior extension of the choroid, continuous with the capsule that encloses the lens, and attaching it to the ciliary muscles.

Figure 1.1 Structures of the eye

Iris

The iris, the most anterior portion of the vascular layer, continuous with the ciliary body, is doughnut-shaped and its central opening, the pupil, appears to be black in color. The iris is composed of rings of muscle fibers, some of which are arranged circularly, contracting to reduce the size of the pupil, with others arranged radially, contracting to increase the size of the pupil, regulating the amount of light admitted to the lens. The iris is suspended in the aqueous space between the cornea and lens, dividing it into anterior and posterior chambers. The larger anterior chamber is between the iris and the cornea, and the posterior chamber is between the lens and the iris. These chambers are filled with the lymph-like aqueous humor, which aids in maintaining the shape of the eyeball, and empties into the canal of Schlemm, an oval channel circling the anterior chamber. The aqueous humor, which is secreted by the ciliary processes, flows through the pupil into the anterior chamber, and the pressure maintained by the balance between secretion and removal of fluid is known as the intraocular pressure.

The reflection of light scattered by pigment substances in the iris results in different colors, with dark eyes having abundant pigment, and blue eyes having less pigment. Some neonates have blue eyes because the pigment does not develop in the stroma (connective tissue fibers forming the major part of the iris) until after birth; however, others have brown eyes at birth because the stromal pigment is already developed.

Lens

The transparent crystalline lens is directly behind the iris of the eye, enclosed in an elastic capsule supported by the suspensory ligament, and focuses the light rays on the retina.

The shape of the lens is altered by the action of ciliary muscles, which affects the refraction (bending) of light rays.

Retina

The innermost of the three coats of the eyeball, the retina, is a soft, delicate membrane that is a contact with, and nourished by, the vascular coat. The retina is the nervous tissue layer with special neuroepithelial cells, the rods and cones, named for their shape, that serve as the photosensitive receptors of light stimuli. The cones are much less numerous than the rods, and are adapted to bright light and color perception as well as for fine details of an object. The rods are much more sensitive for low light vision, but are color blind. Near the center of the back of the retina is a small yellow area called the macula lutea, with a central depression, the fovea centralis, which is the region of clearest vision, in which the cones are most concentrated, and no rods are found. The retina also contains numerous sensory and connector neurons and their process. At a point in the back of the retina, nearer the nose, there is an optic disk, where the nerve fibers from the entire eye converge to form the optic nerve, producing a blind spot because there are no rods or cones present. At the point where the optic nerve pierces the sclera, it is accompanied by the optic central artery and vein, which come from the choroid.

Lacrimal Glands

The lacrimal glands, about the size of an almond kernel, lie under the bones forming the upper, outer orbit, secreting tears which are carried to the conjunctiva by lacrimal ducts. There are several small accessory lacrimal glands lying in fold under the eyelids, which under ordinary circumstances secret sufficient tears to lubricate and clean the eyes, with the main glands called into play only during crying or in response to irritation of the conjunctiva.

The blinking of the eyes spreads the tears over the conjunctival surfaces and directs the fluid into a lacrimal lake at the nasal corner, the inner canthus. The tears are drained from the lake by two small lacrimal ducts that lead into the nose. The opening of the tear ducts into the nose accounts for the "running" of the nose during crying.

The Mechanism of Vision

Vision occurs when light rays enter the pupil and are focused upon the retina by the lens, cornea, and aqueous and vitreous humors. This process of focusing is accomplished by all four components, any of which may develop defects. Light rays from objects 20 feet or more away are relatively parallel and are readily focused on the retina by the normal eye. Closer light rays must be bent more sharply to focus them on the retina. This process, called accommodation, involves an increase in convex curvature of the lens, which is elastic, by ciliary muscle contraction, along with some constriction of the pupil to restrict stray light that might blur the image.

Since both eyes must focus the light rays from an object on corresponding points on the retina to achieve single rather than double vision, the eyeballs are converged by six extrinsic muscles that are attached to the outside of the eyeball and to the bones of the orbit. The slight difference in corresponding points of the retina on which the light rays from the same object are focused, caused by the few inches separating the eyes, as well as the individual's history of visual experiences with near and far objects, accounts for depth perception, or three-dimensionality.

Stimulations of the retinal receptors (rods and cones) are transmitted through the optic nerves to the optic chiasma, then to midbrain areas and the visual cortex areas of the occipital lobe. In the optic chiasma, the optic nerve fibers from the inner (or nasal) half of each retina cross over and join those from the outer (or temporal) half of the retina of the other eye before continuing-on.

Figure 1.2 **Visual fields and pathways**

For example, the fibers from the right half of the left eye link up with those from the right half of the right eye. This accounts for the finding that in conditions producing total loss of nerve transmission in the visual cortex of one hemisphere, there is partial loss of vision in both eyes rather than total loss in either in (Figure 1.2).

Review A

Complete the following:

1. The most important sense organ is the _____ .

2. The mucous membrane covering the exposed third of the eyeball is the _____ .

3. Tears are secreted by _____ glands.

4. There are _____ concentric coats making up the wall of the eyeball.

5. The receptors of light stimuli are the _____ and _____ .

6. The "white of the eye" is called the _____ .

7. Light enters the eye through the transparent part of the eyeball called the _____ .

8. The pigment melanin fills the cells of the _____ .

9. The process by which light rays are bent to focus them on the retina is called _____ .

10. Stimulations of the retinal receptors are transmitted through the optic nerves to the _____ .

THE SENSE OF HEARING

We usually think of the ear as the organ of hearing, which is divided into the external ear, middle ear, and inner ear (oto and auris refer to ear; audi refers to hearing). However, the ear also contains structures responsible for equilibrium.

Structures of the Ear

External Ear

The external ear is made up of the auricle (or pinna, meaning wing), the cartialaginous, cutaneous appendage, and the external auditory meatus (meatus means opening), which is a short, tortuous passage that leads to, and penetrates, the temporal bone. The external auditory canal is entirely lined by skin, and ends blindly at the tympanic membrane (eardrum). Sound waves reach the eardrum through this canal, are picked up by the inner bones of the ear, and transmitted by the auditory nerve to the brain. (Figure 1.3).

Middle Ear

This small, air-filled tympanic cavity in the skull is lined by a mucous membrane and situated between the inner ear and tympanic membrane, communicating through the Eustachian tube with the pharynx. This tube keeps the air pressure equal on both sides of the tympanic membrane, making the air pressure in the middle ear the same as that of the atmosphere. The pharyngeal orifice of the tube is normally closed, but opens during swallowing and yawning, or when a high pressure is created in the nasopharynx, as when blowing the nose or making a forced expiration with the nostrils and mouth closed. The typmpanic membrane is very sensitive to any difference in pressure on its two surfaces, and during rapid changes in altitude, as in airplane ascents and descents, annoying aural effects may be produced, such as ringing sounds in the ears.

In the middle ear there are three tiny connected bones called the auditory ossicles (ossicle means little bone), deriving their names from their shape: the malleus (hammer), the incus (anvil), and the stapes (strirrup). These bones are connected by joints, and bridge the middle ear (tympanic cavity) to transmit sound waves, by the mechanical action of the ossicles, to the inner ear.

Figure 1.3 Structures of the ear

Inner Ear

The inner ear (labyrinth) begins at the oval window, against which the stapes presses, and continues in a labyrinthine cochlea (which means spiral or snail shell shape), which contains three canals that are separated from each other by thin membranes and almost converge at the apex. Two of these canals are bony chambers filled with a perilymph fluid, one of which, the bony vestibular canal, is connected to the oval window that leads to the middle ear. Another, the tympanic canal, is also bony and is connected to the round window opening into the middle ear. The third canal, the cochlear canal, is a membranous chamber filled with endolymph, situated between the other two canals, containing the organ of Corti, a spiral-shaped organ located on the basilar membrane of the cochlear canal, made up of cells with projecting hairs that transmit auditory impulses to the cochlear nerve.

Mechanism of Hearing

Sounds waves enter the external ear and strike the tympanic membrane, causing vibration, which sets into motion the three ossicles, the malleus, the incus, and the stapes, in that order. The stapes is the last to vibrate, and it strikes against the oval window of the vestibular canal, setting into motion the perilymplh fluid in the vestibular and tympanic canals of the cochlea. The vibrating perilymph sets into motion the basilar membrane that separates these two canals, thereby disturbing the endolympph fluid in the membranous area of the cochlea. Hair cells of the organ of Corti, located in this area, are stimulated by the movement of the endolymph, and by bending against another membrane (the tectorial), the hair cells transmit the impulse to the brain by way of the auditory nerve. The final interpretation of sound is made by the brain.

Sense of Equilibrium

In addition to the structures just described, there are three semicircular canals in the labyrinth that lie in planes at right angles to each other, plus a utricle, and a saccule in each inner ear. These are the structures of equilibrium. (See Figure 1.3).

The saccule and utricle are small sacs that are lined with sensitive hairs and contain particles, called otoliths (lith refers to stone), that are made up of calcium carbonate. The otoloiths press on the hair cells through the pull of gravity and stimulate the initiation of impulses from the hair cells to the brain through their basal sensory nerve fibers. The utricles and saccules, which together are called the vestibule, are responsible for the reactions that result from position change and change of rectilinear motion (movement in a straight line).

The semicircular canals, which are liquid-filled, respond to rotary, or turning, movement. They are positioned at right angles to each other, each corresponding to one of the three spatial planes. Turning the head in any direction stimulates at least one of the canals. Inside each canal are hair cell receptors that bend in response to rotary motion, stimulating nerve fibers that carry impulses to the vestibular branch of the auditory nerve, and then to the brain.

Review B

Complete the following:

1. The ear has two functions: and _____

2. The tympanic membrane is also known as the _____ .

3. The _____ equalizes air pressure on both sides of the tympanic membrane.

4. The inner ear has a labyrinthine cochlea which contains _____ canals.

5. The three ossicles are the _____ , and _____ .

6. The external auditory canal is entirely lined by _____ .

7. The stapes presses against the _____ .

8. Hair cells transmit sound stimulation to the brain by way of the _____ nerve.

9. The _____ membrane separates the vestibular and tympanic canals of the cochlea.

10. The structures of equilibrium are three _____ plus a _____ and a _____ .

THE SENSE OF SMELL

Smell is one of the most primitive senses. In many animals it is very acute and of paramount importance because it serves to warn the animal of approaching enemies, guides it in its quest for food, and even motivates the sex reflexes. In humans it also serves to warn of the danger. Smoke is often smelled before the fire is located; escaping gas from a leaky burner or pipeline can be smelled before a person is overcome or carelessly lights the match that causes an explosion.

The peripheral organ for smell is the nose (naso and rhino refer to nose), with its external parts and nasal cavities. The organ of smell is the olfactory epithelium of the nose, and odor is perceived through stimulation of its cells. The olfactory (olfact refers to smell) receptors are confined to the nasal mucosa over a relatively small area in a narrow niched formed by the superior nasal concha (concha means shell-shaped), the upper part of the septum (wall between the two nasal cavities), and the root of the nose. **(Figure 1-4)**

The root of the nose is the upper, narrow end between the eyes, and the bridge of the nose is the part that extends from the root to the tip (apex). The external nares (nostrils) are the two oval openings separated from one another by the lower part of the septum, and the flexible lower portions on each side bordering the nostrils are the alae (ala is the singular form and means wing-like).

The nose is formed by the nasal bones and cartilage. The nasal bones are the turbinates, superior (upper), medial (middle), and inferior (lower) conchae. Nasal cartilages are connected to each other and to the bones by fibrous tissue. Just inside the nasal cavities is a lining of skin with a ring of coarse hairs, whose function is to trap dust and foreign particles during inspiration. The mucous membrane lining the nose is continuous with particular connecting areas, and infections of this membrane are easily spread to them. These connecting areas include the nasopharynx, the Eustachian tube (auditory canal), the middle ear cavity, the sphenoidal, ethmoidal, frontal, and maxillary sinuses, and the palatine bones and tear ducts.

The stimulation of the olfactory epithelium is initially transmitted to the olfactory bulb, and from there continues on to the olfactory centers in the brain. Six basic odors have been identified, interacting with each other to produce the variety we experience: flowery, fruity, spicy, resinous, burned, and putrid. The sense of smell is far more sensitive than the sense of taste, and complements it, as is evident when a respiratory infection blocks the sense of smell, causing food to lose its customary flavors.

THE SENSE OF TASTE

The organs of taste in humans are the taste buds, located mainly in the papillae (small projections) on the tongue, but a few many be found in the mucous membrane that covers the soft palate, the fauces (opening from the mouth to the pharynx) and the epiglottis.

The sense of taste is limited to four primary, or fundamental, tastes: sweet, sour (acid), salt, and bitter. The various other tastes that we experience are blends of these. For a substance to arouse a sensation of taste, it must be dissolved either in solution or by the saliva, which accounts for the location of the taste buds on a moist surface. Many substances that we think we taste are, in reality, only smelled, and their taste depends upon their odor. For this reason smell is sometimes described as "taste at a distance"

(Figure 1.4) Olfactory centers in the brain

Review C

Complete the following:

1. The five special senses are _____, _____, _____, _____, _____.

2. The _____ of the nose is the organ of smell.

3. Another term for nostrils is _____.

4. There are _____ basic odors.

5. Stimulation of the organ of smell is initially transmitted to the olfactory _____.

6. The organs of taste are located mainly on the _____.

7. The organs of taste are the _____.

8. There are _____ fundamental tastes.

9. Taste depends on _____.

10. To arouse a sensation of taste a substance must be _____.

TOUCH AND OTHER CUTANEOUS SENSES

The skin is a receptor for the sensations of touch as well as those of heat, cold, and pain (Figure 1.5) Touch (also called light pressure) is experienced as a function of stimulation of free sensory nerve endings (dendrites) everywhere in the skin, but especially around hair follicles. Tactile corpuscles in the epidermis called Merkel's disks relay light touch and superficial pressure, and other structures in the corium (layer below the epidermis) called Meissner's corpuscles are believed to medicate light pressure sensations. Heavier pressure stimulates the Pacinian corpuscles, which are lamellated (layered) bodies of sensory nerve tissue located in the subcutaneous layer.

Thermal sensations of heat and cold are experienced in response to changes of even a few degrees from skin temperature, but the precise mechanisms are not known. Free nerve endings are believed to be the main receptors, along with Ruffinian corpuscles, which are sensory end structures located in the corium. Also considered as mediators of heat and cold are the capillaries of the skin (Figure 1.5)

Pain sensations have not been linked to any specific nerve structures, but are believed to be transmitted by free sensory nerve endings found just below the surface of the skin.

The skin areas of the body have varying sensitivities to sensation as a function of the distributions of receptors in the differing areas. The most sensitive areas generally are those most involved in obtaining information about one-self and the external world, such as the lips and fingers, whereas fewer receptors are found on the back of the hand or the dorsal surfaces.

(Figure 1.5) Sensory receptors

Table 1.1

THE SPECIAL SENSES

Sense	Organ	Receptors	Stimulus
Sight(vision)	Retina of eye	Rods(120 million/eye) Wavelengths of light Cones (8 million/eye)	
Hearing (audition)	basilar membrane of Cochlea (inner ear) of Corti	Hair cells of the organ vibrations	Sound
Balance (equilibrium)	Utricle, saccule, and Hair cells Semicircular canals of Inner ear	Mechanical and fluid pressure	
Smell (olfaction)	Mucous membranes of Upper nasal cavity	Olfactory epithelium hair cells (60 million)	Chemical gas
Taste (gustation)	Surface of tongue	Taste buds on papillae (10,000)	Dissolved chemicals
Touch pressure	Layers of skin	Free nerve endings, Meissner's corpuscles Pacinian corpuscles, Merkel's disks	Mechanical pressure
Pain		Free nerve endings	High Intensity of stimuli
Warmth, cold		Free nerve endings, Rufflan corpuscles, Skin capillaries	Thermal energy

Review D

Complete the following:

1. The skin is a receptor for _____, _____, and _____.

2. Stimulation of free sensory nerve endings produces the sense of _____.

3. The most sensitive skin areas are _____ the and _____.

4. The least sensitive skin areas are the _____ surfaces.

5. The Pacinian corpuscles are stimulated by _____ pressure.

Answers to Review Questions: The Special Senses

Review A

1. Eye

2. Conjucnctiva

3. Lacrimal

4. Three

5. Rods and cones

6. Sclera

7. Cornea

8. Choroid

9. Accommodation

10. Optic chiasma

Review B

1. Hearing and equilibrium

2. Eardrum

3. Eustachian tube

4. Three

5. Malleus, incus, stapes

6. Skin

7. Oval window

8. Auditory

9. Basilar

10. Semicircular canals, utricle, saddule

Review C

1. Vision, hearing, smell, taste, touch

2. Olfactory epithelium

3. External nares or nostrils

4. Six

5. Bulb

6. Tongue

7. Taste buds

8. Four

9. Odor

10. Dissolved

Review D

1. Touch, heat, cold, and pain

2. Touch/pain

3. Lips and fingers

4. Dorsal

5. Heavy/heavier

Chapter 09 Exercises

THE SPEICAL SENSES: THE SOURCES OF INFORMATION

Exercise 1: Complete the following:

1. The peripheral organ for smell is the _____.

2. The upper narrow end of the nose between the eyes is called the _____.

3. The structures that constitute the essential part of the eye are the _____ and the _____.

4. The movement of opening the eye is a function of the _____.

5. The anterior, transparent portion of the fibrous coat of the eyeball, through which light enters the eye is the _____.

6. The part between the sclera and retina whose posterior part is a thin membrane with a vascular layer is the _____.

7. The innermost of the three coats of the eyeball, constituting the nervous layer on which light rays are focus is the _____.

8. The divisions of the ear are the _____, _____, and _____.

9. The malleus, incus, and stapes perform the important function of _____.

10. The structures of equilibrium are the _____, _____, and _____.

Exercise 2: Using the list of terms below, identify each part in Figure 1.6 by writing the name in the corresponding blank.

Vitreous chamber	1. _____
Conjunctiva	2. _____
Lens	3. _____
Retina	4. _____
Iris	5. _____
Sclera	6. _____
Aqueous chamber	7. _____
Optic nerve	8. _____
Cornea	9. _____
Ciliary processes	10. _____
Choroid	11. _____

Pupil   12. _____
Ciliary muscle   13. _____
Suspensory ligament   14. _____

(Figure 1.6) Structures of the eye

(Figure 1.7)

Exercise 3: Using the list of terms below, identify each part in Figure 1.7 by writing the name in the corresponding blank.

Temporal bone   1. _____
Tympanic cavity   2. _____
Auditory nerve   3. _____
Pinna   4. _____
Cochlea   5. _____
Incus   6. _____
Mastoid process   7. _____
Eustachian tube   8. _____
Tympanic membrane   9. _____
External auditory meatus or canal   10. _____
Malleus   11. _____
Stapes   12. _____
Semicircular canals   13. _____
Styloid process   14. _____

Exercise 4: Matching:

1. The depressed area in the center of the back of the retina, the area of clearest vision
   _____

2. Angles at the ends of the slits between the eyelids _____

3. Specialized outer ends of the visual cells in the retina that are adapted to bright light, acute vision, and color perception _____

4. Special cylindrical neuroepithelial cells in the retina, highly sensitive to low light
   _____

5. The partition separating the external nares _____

6. Special organ of hearing located on basilar membrane of the cochlea _____

7. The projecting posterior part of the ear that lies outside the head _____

8. Structures for equilibrium in the labyrinth _____

9. Structure leading from the ear to the throat _____

10. Structure that separates the middle ear from the external ear _____

A. Eustachian tube   F. Tympanic membrane
B. Canthi   G. Septum
C. Rods   H. Fovea
D. Semicircular canals I. pinna
E. Cones   J. organ of Corti

Exercise 5: In the blank following each pair of words, indicate whether their meaning is the same or different.

1. Inner ear
    Labyrinth   _____

2. Auricle
    External nares   _____

3. Tympanic membrane
    Eardrum   _____

4. Eyelid
    Palpebral   _____

5. Earwax
    Cerumen   _____

Exercise 6: Give the meaning of the components in the following words and then define the word as a whole. Suffixes meaning pertaining to or state or condition shown following a slash mark (/), are not to be defined separately. Before reaching for your medical dictionary, check the glossary at the end of the chapter.

1. Blepharitis:
    Blephar
    itis

2. Diplopia:
    Dipl
    Op/ia

3. Nyctalopia:
   Nyct
   Al
   Op/ia

4. Retinoblastoma:
   Retino
   Blast
   Oma

5. Dacryoadenectomy:
   Dacryo
   Aden
   Ectomy

6. Eustachitis:
   Eustach
   Itis

7. Myringitis
   Myring
   Itis

8. Tympanomastoiditis:
   Tympano
   Mastoid
   Itis

9. Xerophthalmus:
   Xer
   Ophthalm/us

10. Otalgia:
    Ot
    Algia

11. Dacryocystistis:
    Dacryo
    Cyst
    Itis

12. Ageusia:
    A
    Geus/ia

13. Otorrhea:

    Oto

    Neur

    Itis

14. Optic neuritis:

    Op/tic

    Neur

    Itis

15. Retinitis:

    Retin

    Itis

RESEARCH GUIDE

Research Guide

Name _____ **Period** _____

Research question(s) _____

_____

Search terms _____

Note taking

Publishing information	
Title	
Author	
Company	
Date	
Web page/sponsor	
Web address	

PAPER FORMAT

Paper Format

Below are some basic guideline for formatting a paper in MLA style.

General Guidelines

- Type your paper on a computer and print it out on standard, white 8.5 x 11—inch paper.

- Double-space the text of your paper, and use a legible font (e.g. Times New Roman). Whatever font you choose, MLA recommends that the regular and italics type styles contrast enough that they are recognizable one from another. The font size should be 12 pt.

- Leave only one space after periods or other punctuation marks (unless otherwise instructed by your instructor).

- Set the margins of your document to 1 inch on all sides.

- Indent the first line of paragraphs one half—inch from the left margin. MLA recommends that you use the Tab key as opposed to pushing the Space Bar five times.

- Create a header that numbers all pages consecutively in the upper right-hand corner, one-half from the top and flush with the right margin. (Note: Your instructor may ask that you omit the number on your first page. Always follow your instructor's guidelines.)

- Use italics throughout your essay for the titles of longer works and, only when absolutely necessary, providing emphasis.

- If you have any endnotes, include them on a separate page before your Works Cited page. Entitle the section Notes (centered, unformatted).

- Formatting the First Page of Your Paper

- Do not make a title page for your paper unless specifically requested.

- In the upper left-hand corner of the first page, list your name, your instructor's name, the course, and the date. Again, be sure to use double-spaced text.

- Double space again and center the title. Do not underline, italicize, or place your title in quotation marks; write the title in Title Case(standard capitalization), not in all capital letters.

- Use quotation marks and/or italics when referring to other works in your title, just as you would in your text: Fear and Loathing in Las Vegas as Morality Play; Human Weariness in "After Apple Picking"

- Double space between the title and the first line of the text.

- Create a header in the upper right-hand corner that includes your last name, followed by a space with a page number; number all pages consecutively with Arabic numerals (1, 2, 3, 4, etc.), one-half inch from the top and flush with the right margin. (Note: Your instructor or other readers may ask that you omit last name/page number header on your first page. Always follow instructor guidelines.)

CREATING A WORKS CITED PAGE

CREATING A WORKS CITED PAGE

GENERAL INFORMATION

Works Cited and Bibliography are not the same. In Works Cited you only list items you have actually cited. In a Bibliography you list all the material you have consulted in preparing your essay whether or not you have actually cited the work.

1. DO NOT number entries

2. DO NOT list sources separately by categories. All references are placed in ONE ALPHABETICAL LIST by first word, regardless of where it came from.

3. Begin on a new page. Start on the 6th line from the top (or 1" down from the top of the paper), center, and type the following title: Bibliography. Double space after the title. List all entries in alphabetical order by the first word, taking into consideration the rules governing titles that begin with articles.

4. Begin the first line of each entry flush at the left margin. Keep trying until you run out of room at the end of the line. Indent 5 spaces for second and subsequent lines of the same entry. Double-space all lines, both within and between entries.

Sample

Works Cited
Didion, Joan. The Year of Magical Thinking. New York: Knopf, 2005
Emiliano Zapata. Encyclopedia of World Biography. Ed Paula K.
Byers. Vol. 16 2nd ed. Detroit: Gale, 1998. P489-490. 23vols

Basic MLA Guide

<u>Books</u>

Author(s). Title of Book. Place of Publication: Publisher, Year of Pulication.

<u>Book with one author-Sample</u>

Henley, Patricia. The Hummingbird House. Denver: MacMurray, 1999

<u>Book with a corporate author-Sample</u>

American Allergy Association. Allergies in Children. New York: Random, 1998.

<u>BOOK OR ARTICLE WITH NO AUTHOR NAMED</u>

<u>Title.</u> Place of Publication: Publisher, Year of Publication.

<u>Book or article with no author-Sample</u>

<u>Encyclopedia of Indiana.</u> New York: Somerset, 1993.

"Cigarette Sales Fall 30 % as California Tax Rises." <u>New York Times</u> 14 Sept. 1999:A17.

<u>AN ARTICLE IN A PERIODICAL (SUCH AS A NEWSPAPER OR MAGAZINE)</u>

Author (s). "Title of Article." Title of Source Day Month Year: pages.

<u>Poniewozik, James. "TV Makes a Too-Close Call." Time 20 Nov. 2000: 70-71</u>

<u>A WEB SITE</u>

Author (s). Name of Page. Date of Posting/Revision. Name of institution/organization affiliated with the site. Date of Access < electronic address>.

<u>Web site examples</u>

Felluga. Dino. <u>Undergraduate Guide to Literary Theory</u>. 17 Dec. 1999 Purdue University. 15 Nov.

2000. <u>Purdue Online Writing Lab</u>. 2003.

Purdue University. 10 Feb. 2003 <u>http://owl.english.purdue.edu</u>.

AN ARTICLE IN AN ONLINE JOURNAL OR MAGAZINE

Author (s). "Title of Article." Title of Journal Volume. Issue (Year):

Pages/Paragraphs. Date of Access <electronic address>

AN ARTICLE OR PUBLICATION RETRIEVED FROM AN ELECTRONIC DATABASE

Author. "Title of Article." Publication Name Volume Number (if necessary)

Publication Date: page number-page number. Database name. Service name. Library Name, City, State. Date of access <electronic address of the database>.

Electronic Database example Smith, Martin. "World Domination for Dummies." Journal of Despotry Feb. 2000: 66-72. Expanded Academic ASAP. Gale Group Databases.

Purdue University Libraries, West Lafayette, IN. 19 February 2003

http://www.infotrac.galegroup.com

January 25, 2003

Mr. E. B. Burns
Director of Nurses
St. Joseph's Hospital
P.O. Bos 123
Los Angeles, CA 90880

Dear Mr. Burns:

I am responding to your advertisement in Nurses World on January 14, 2003. I am interested in applying for the position of nurse assistant. I graduated from Medical Technologies High School on Decemeber 15, 2002. I studied nursing assisting and am well qualified for this position. My course work included communication, CPR, and a core of courses that prepared me to be employed as a nursing assistant. I also worked in a hospital setting eight hours a week for sixteen weeks. My attendance is excellent, and I am very reliable. My goal is to use my skills a nursing assistant and to be an exemplary employee.

My resume is enclosed. Also included is a list of skills I have mastered. I know that I am well qualified for this position. I am looking forward to an opportunity to interview for this position. I will call on Monday, February 3, at 9:00 a.m. and hope to arrange an interview at that time.

I you require additional information, or want to contact me, please call me at (123) 456-7890 after 3:00 p.m.

Sincerely,

Mark Adams, CNA

Mary Jane Rodgers

800 N. Euclid
New York, New York 00333
Home: 220-666-8340
Message: 220-620-9180

Career Plans:

Complete 2—year Associate of Science Nursing Program
Short-range: Nursing assistant
Long-range: Complete a Bachelor of Science Program as a registered nurse

Experience:

2002-present Henry's Hamburger Shop New York, NY
Sales Clerk

- Food preparation

- Counting inventory

- Customer Service

- Operating a cash register and making change

- Maintaining health standards

200-2002 June Allison New York, Ny
Babysitter

- Meal preparation

- Overnight care of two children, 8 and 10 years of age

- Planning recreation

Family

Responsibilities

- Prepare dinner 2-3 times a week

- Weekly gardening

- Perform minor household tasks

Experience

Diploma candidate 2003 Hoover High School

Interests

Dancing, classical music, reading, skiing, member of Explorer Scouts Medical Post and Health Occupation

Students of America

Skills and Strengths

Fluent in oral and written Spanish communication
Proficient in Windows programs including Word, WordPerfect, Excel and Lotus applications
table 1.2

888 Whitegate Avenue
Los Angeles, CA 90820

February 10, 2003

Mr. E. B. Burns
Director of Nurses
St. Joseph's Hospital
P.O. Box 123
Los Angeles, CA 90880

Dear Mr. Burns:

Thank you for interviewing me yesterday afternoon. The position interests me very much, and I know that I will do a good job for you. I hope that you will give me an opportunity to work for the nursing department at St. Joseph's.

Sincerely,

Mark Adams, CNA

table 1.3

JOB INTERVIEW TIPS

Job Interview Tips

Preparation:

- Learn about the organization.

- Have a specific job or jobs in mind.

- Review your qualifications for the job.

- Prepare answers to broad questions about your self

- Review your resume

- Practice an interview with a friend or relative.

- Arrive before the scheduled time of your interview.

Personal Appearance:

- Be well groomed.

- Dress appropriately.

- Do not chew gum or smoke.

The Interview:

- Answer each question concisely.

- Respond promptly.

- Use good manners. Learn the name of your interviewer and shake hands as you meet.

- Use proper English and avoid slang.

- Be cooperative and enthusiastic.

- Ask questions about the position and the organization.

- Thank the interviewer, and follow up with the letter.

Test (if the employer gives one):

- **Listen closely to instructions.**

- **Read each question carefully.**

- **Write legibly and clearly.**

- **Budget your time wisely, and don't dwell on one question.**

Information to Bring to an interview:

- **Social Security number**

- **Driver's license number**

- **Resume. Although not all employers require applicants to bring a resume, you should be able to furnish the interviewer with information about your education, training, and previous employment.**

- **Usually an employer requires three references. Get permission from people before using their names, and make sure they will give you a good reference. Try to avoid using relatives. For each reference, provide the following information: Name, address, telephone number, and job title.**

Identify the Problem:

Identify possible solutions (Generate as many potential solutions as you can.):

1.

2.

3.

4.

5.

Pick the Best Solution:

Defend your Solution (Explain why you have chosen the solution, why is it best?):

Evaluate the outcome of your problem based on the solution you have chosen:

Introduction to Microsoft PowerPoint

Objectives:

Lesson 1-Microsoft PowerPoint Tour

- **Define Multimedia Presentation**
- **Recognize parts of the screen**
- **Create a blank presentation**
- **Create a presentation from a template**
- **Adjust PowerPoint views**
- **Change the theme**

Lesson 2—Microsoft PowerPoint Basics

- **Insert a slide**
- **Change a slide layout**
- **Insert and format Clip Art**
- **Insert and format graphics**
- **Insert and adjust audio clips**
- **Insert photographs from a file**
- **Move and resize pictures**
- **Perform spell checking**

Lesson 3—Effective Presentations

- **Describe several tips used to create effective presentations**

Student Prerequisites

- **Microsoft Office Fundamentals module**

Teacher Preparation

- Students will be downloading and working with Microsoft application files. At the beginning of each lesson, students are instructed to save these files to a location indicated by the teacher. Make sure students know where the files are to be stored prior to starting the lessons.

- Students will be creating many documents. The total number of documents for the class can be large because each student typically create one document per lesson. You need to decide how to assess these documents. There are many options such as giving a checkmark for completion, grading only one of the documents, or not assessing any of the documents and just relying on the quizzes and/or module test for the unit grade. When you have decided on an option make sure to communicate it to the students.

- Each lesson has at least one Challenge task towards the end of the lesson that extends one or more of the objective covered in the lesson. Because they are extensions they are not necessarily required. You should review the Challenge task and determine the "rules" or reasons students should either complete or skip them.

Time Required for Lessons
28 to 33 minutes. Times will vary depending on the age and experience of the learner.

Lesson Description
Lesson 1—Microsoft PowerPoint Tour

Students will take a virtual tour of Microsoft PowerPoint. They will learn the basics of creating blank presentations and presentations from a template. Students will also learn how to change power point views and change a presentations' theme.

Lesson 2—Microsoft Power Point Basics

Students will gain experience in PowerPoint by finishing a simple presentation to help their family choose a vacation destination. Completing the presentation requires insertion and formating of clip art, photographs and audio clips.

Students will be required to download an attachment from the lesson.

This lesson includes two Challenge tasks, which gives students the opportunity to spend more time working on things they have learned.

Lesson 3—Effective Presentations

Students will learn about 10 tips to create more effective presentations and use some of those tips to improve an existing presentation.

Students will be required to download an attachment from the lesson.

This lesson includes a Challenge task, which gives students the opportunity to spend more time working on things they have learned.

Lesson 1-Enter Data

- **Identify types of data.**

- **Enter Data.**

Lesson 2-Format Data

- **Change font formatting**

- **Apply number formats.**

Lesson 3—Delete & Copy Data

- **Delete cell contents**

- **Cut, copy, and paste data.**

- **AutoFill cell contents.**

Lesson 4-Make Corrections

- **Find and replace data.**

- **Check for spelling errors.**

Lesson 5-Assignment

- **Apply concepts learned in the lessons to a working document.**

Prerequisites

- **Microsoft Office Basics, Unit 1—Common Features**

- **Microsoft Office Basics, Unit 2-Working with Files**

- **Spreadsheets: Basic, Unit 1—Introduction to Spreadsheets**

Recommended Student Tasks

1. **View online content**

2. **Answer lesson questions**

3. **Complete the assignment**

Assignment

Prerequisites:

- **Lesson 1—Enter Data**

- **Lesson 2—Format Data**

- **Lesson 3-Delete & Copy Data**

- **Lesson 4-Make Corrections**

Materials:

- **Microsoft ® Excel**

CHAPTER 11

THE HIPAA PRIVACY STANDARDS

Chapter 11

The HIPPA Privacy Standards

Figure 2-1

Documentation Ex ample

Ribielli, James E.

5/19/2014

CHIEF COMPLAINT: This 79-year old male presents with sudden and extreme weakness. He got up from a seated position and became light-headed.

PAST MEDICAL HISTORY: History of congestive heart failure, on multiple medications, including Cardizem, Enalapril 5mg qd, and Lasix 40 mg qd.

PHYSICAL EXAMINATION: No postural change in blood pressure. BP, 114/61 with a pulse of 49, sitting: BP, 111/56 with a pulse 50, stands. Patient denies being light-headed at this time.

HEENT: Unremarkable.

NECK: Supple without jugular or venous distension.

LUNGS: Clear to auscultation and percussion.

HEART: S1 and S2 normal; no systolic or diastolic murmurs; no S3, S4. No dysrhythmia.

ABDOMEN: Soft without organomegaly, mass, or bruit.

EXTREMITIES: Unremarkable. Pulses strong and equal.

LABORATORY DATA: Hemoglobin, 12.3 White count, 10.800. Normal Electrolytes. ECG shows sinus bradycardia.

DIAGNOSIS: Weakness on the basis of sinus bradycardia, probably Cardizem induced.

TREATMENT: Patient told to change positions slowly when moving from sitting to standing, and from lying to standing.

For Privacy of Individually Identifiable Health Information rule is known as the HIPPA Privacy Rule. Enacted on April 14, 2003, the HIPAA privacy standards were the first comprehensive federal protection for the privacy of health information. These national standards protect individuals' medical records and other personal health information. Before the HIPPA Privacy Rule became law, the personal information stored in hospitals, physician practices, and health plans were governed by a patchwork of federal and state laws. Some state laws were strict, but others were not.

The Privacy Rule says that covered entities must:

- Have privacy policies and procedures that are appropriate for their health care services

- Notify patients about their privacy rights and how their information can be used or disclosed

- Train employees so that they understand the privacy practices

- Appoint a privacy official responsible for seeing that the privacy policies and procedures are implemented

- Safeguard patients' records

COMPLIANCE TIP

Privacy Officers

The privacy official at a small physician practice may be the office manager, who also has other duties. At a large health plan, the position of privacy official may be full-time.

Table 2-1 Advantages of Electronic Medical Records

Immediate access to Health information	The EMR is simultaneously accessible to all qualified users. Compared to sorting through papers in a paper folder, an EMR database can save time when vital patient information is needed. Once information is updated in a patient record, it is available to all who need access, whether across the hall or across town.
Computerized physician Order management	Physicians can enter orders for prescriptions, test, and other services at any time, along with the patients' diagnosis.
Clinical decision support	An EMR system can provide access to approved medical websites with the latest medical research to help medical decision making

Automated alerts and Reminders

The system can provide the staff with medical alerts and reminders to ensure that patients are scheduled for regular screenings and other preventive practices. Alerts can also be created to identify patient safety issues, such as possible drug interactions.

Electronic communication

An EMR system can provide a means of secure an easily accessible communication between physicians and staff and in some offices between physicians and patients.

Patient support

Some EMR programs allow patients to access Their medical records and request appointments. These programs also offer patient education on health topics and instructions on preparing for common medical tests, such as HDL cholesterol tests.

Administration and Reporting

The EMR may include administrative tools, including reporting systems that enable facilities And state reporting requirements.

Error reduction

An EMR can decrease medical errors that result from illegible chart notes, since notes are entered electronically on a computer or a handheld device.

Thinking It Through

In addition to electronic medical records that are used in medical offices and hospitals, many health care industry and government officials are encouraging the development of personal health records. An article from Family Practice Management(13, 5 (May 2006): 57-62; www.aaafg.org/fpm/20060500/57anin.html)related the way a PHR was used:

Meet Mrs. Johnson, a 79 year-old with diabetes, congestive heart failure and an electronic personal health record (PHR).

Mrs. Johnson saw her family physician this morning, and on the way home she realized she had already forgotten his instructions for her new heart medication. Was it two pills once a day, or did he say one pill twice a day? She also wondered when she would find out the results of the blood test he had ordered to determine her potassium level, which she struggles to keep normal. She was worried but knew that her online personal health record would enable her to find the answer to both questions as soon as she arrived home.

Once there, Mrs. Johnson sat down at her computer and logged in to the personal health record Web site that her family physician offered his patients. First, she sent a secure e-mail to her physician asking how to take her new medication. She was impressed to see that the new heart drug already was on her medication list. Next, Mrs. Johnson checked her in-box, where a message from her physician was waiting. Mrs. Johnson opened the message and was relieved to read that her potassium test had come back normal. Finally, she browsed the site's patient-education area and printed an article on potassium-rich diets before signing off.

The personal health record had informed and educated Mrs. Johnson. It also had saved her and her doctor's office from one or two follow-up phone calls. But its most important benefit on this day was still to come.

That evening, Mrs. Johnson woke with severe chest pain and shortness of breath. She was able to dial 911 and was rushed to the hospital. The emergency department physician diagnosed an acute coronary syndrome and started to write Mrs. Johnson's admission orders. He asked what medications she was taking. She could not remember all of them but told him that her entire medical record was available on the Internet. She gave him the password, which the physician used to access her online personal health record. There he found her medication list and her medication allergies, which included an aspirin allergy. He canceled the aspirin order he had just written included an aspirin allergy. He canceled the aspirin order he had just written and switched it to clopidogrel, signing, "a potential adverse drug event avoided, thanks to patient's PHR."

Based on this patient's history, what advantages can you cite for the use of PHR's? Are there any drawbacks to their use?

The HIPPAA Privacy Rule covers the use and disclosure of patients' protected health information (PHI). PHI is defined as individually identifiable health information that is transmitted or maintained by electronic media, such as over the Internet, or transmitted maintained in any other form or medium. This information includes a person's:

- Name

- Address (including street address, city, county, ZIP code)

- Relatives' and employers' names

- Birth date

- Telephone numbers

- Fax number

- E-mail address

- Social Security number

- Medical record number

- Health plan beneficiary number

- Account number

- Certificate or license number

- Serial number of any vehicle or other device

- Website address

- Fingerprints or voiceprints

- Photographic images

Minimum Necessary Standard

When using or disclosing protected health information, a covered entity must try to limit the information to the minimum amount of PHI necessary for the intended purpose. The minimum necessary standard means taking reasonable safeguards to protect PHI from being accidentally released to those not needing the information during a correct use or disclosure.

Designated Record Set

Also, the covered entity only must release a designated record set, not all information. For purposes of the HIPAA Privacy Rule, record means any item, collection, or grouping of information that includes PHI and is maintained by a covered entity. The HIPAA term for a group of records is a designated record set (DRS). For a provider, the designated record set means the medical and billing records the provider maintains. It does not include appointment and surgery schedules, requests for lab tests, and birth and death records. It also does not include mental health information, psychotherapy notes, and genetic information, which are protected by more stringent release guidelines. For a health plan, the designated record set includes enrollment, payment, claim decisions, and medical management systems of the plan.

Notice of Privacy Practices(NPP)

Covered entities must state their policies and procedures in a document called the Notice of Privacy Practices (NPP). They must also make their NPP's available on request to any person who requests them. If the CE is a health care provider with a physical service delivery site, it must have the notice available at the site for individuals to take with them.

CEs must also give each patient a Notice of Privacy Practices at the first contact or encounter. For example, health plans must comply with specific requirements for notifying enrollees in their plans.

To meet this requirement, physician practices give patients their NPPs. The notice explains how patients PHI may be used and describes their rights. Practices may choose to use a layered approach to giving patients the notice. On top of the information packet is a short notice, like the one shown in Figure 2.2 that briefly describes the uses and disclosures of PHI and the person's rights. The longer notice is placed beneath it.

If the first service delivery to an individual is electronic, the CE must provide the electronic notice automatically in response to the individual's first request for service. For example, the first time an individual requests a refill of a prescription through a covered Internet pharmacy, the pharmacy must respond with the pharmacy's Notice of Privacy Practices. Individuals who receive electronic notices have the right to obtain paper copies on request.

Figure 2-2: Example of a Notice of Privacy Practices

ABC Clinic Notice of Privacy Practices

THIS NOTICE DESCRIBES HOW MEDICAL INFORMATION ABOUT YOU MAY BE USED AND DISCLOSED AND HOW YOU CAN GET ACCESS TO THIS INFORMATION, PLEASE REVIEW IT CAREFULLY.

WHY ARE YOU GETTING THIS NOTICE?

ABC Clinic is required by federal and state law to maintain the privacy of your health information. The use and disclosure of your health information is governed by regulations under the Health Insurance Portability and Accountability Act of 1996 (HIPPA) and the requirements of applicable state law. For health information covered by HIPAA, we are required to provide you

with this Notice, please contact our Privacy Officer at 877-555-1313. We will ask you to sign an "acknowledgment" indicating that you have been provided with this notice

WHAT HEALTH INFORMATION IS PROTECTED?

We are committed to protecting the privacy of information we gather about you while providing health-related services. Some examples of protected health information are:

- Information indicating that you are a patient receiving treatment or other health-related services from our physicians or staff;

- Information about your health condition (such as a disease you may have);

- Information about health care products or services you have received or may receive in the future (such as an operation); or

- Information about your health care benefits under an insurance plan (such as whether a prescription is covered); when combined with:

- Demographic information (such as your name, address, or insurance status);

- Unique numbers that may identify you (such as your Social Security number, your phone number or your driver's license number); and

- Other types of information that may identify who you are.

SUMMARY OF THIS NOTICE

This summary includes references to paragraphs throughout this notice that you may read for additional information

1. **Written Authorization Requirement**. We may use your health information or share it with others in order to treat your condition, obtain payment for that treatment, and run our business operations. We generally need your written authorization for other uses and disclosures of your health information, unless an exception described in this Notice applies.

2. **Authorizing Transfer of Your Records**. You may request that we transfer your records to another person or organization by completing a written authorization form. This form will specify what information is being released, to whom, and for what purpose. The authorization will have an expiration date.

3. **Canceling Your Written Authorization**. If you provide us with written authorization, you may revoke, or cancel it any time, except to the extent that we have already relied upon it. To revoke a written authorization, please write to the doctor's office where you initially gave your authorization.

4. **Exceptions to Written Authorization Requirement**. There are some situations in which we do not need your written authorization before using your health information or sharing it with others. They include: . . . . *Treatment, Payment, and Operations.* As mentioned above, we may use your health information or share it with others in order to treat your condition, obtain payment for that treatment, and run our business operations . . . . . . *Family and Friends.* If you do not object, we will share information about your health with family and friends involved in your care . . . . . *Research.* Although we will generally try to obtain your written authorization before using your health information for research purposes, there may be certain situations in which we are not required to obtain your written authorization . . . . . . *De-identified Information.* We may use or disclose your health information if we have removed any information that might identify you. When all identifying information is removed, we say that the health information is "completely de-identified." We may also use and disclose "partially de-identified" information if the person who will receive it agrees in writing to protect your privacy when using the information . . . . . *Incidental Disclosures.* We may inadvertently use or disclose your health information despite having taken all reasonable precautions to protect the privacy and confidentiality of your health information . . . . . . *Emergencies or Public Need.* We may use or disclose your health information in an emergency or for important public health needs. For example, we may share your information with public health officials at the state or city health departments who are authorized to investigate and control the spread of diseases.

5. **How to Access Your Health Information**. You generally have the right to inspect and get copies of your health information.

6. **How to Correct Your Health Information** you have the right to request that we amend your health information if you believe it is inaccurate or incomplete.

7. **How to Identify Others Who Have Received Your Health Information**. You have the right to receive an "accounting of disclosures." This is a report that identifies certain persons or organizations to which we have disclosed your health information. All disclosures are made according to the protections described in this Notice of Privacy Practices. Many routine disclosures we make (for treatment, payment, or business operations among others) will not be included in this report. However, it will identify many non-routine disclosures of your information.

8. **How to Request Additional Privacy Protections**. You have the right to request further restrictions on the way we use your health information or share it with others. However, we are not required to agree to the restriction you request. If we do agree with your request, we will be bound by our agreement.

9. **How to Request Alternative Communications**. You have the right to request that we contact you in a way that is more confidential for you, such as at home instead of at work. We will try to accommodate all reasonable requests.

10. **How Someone May Act on your Behalf.** You have the right to name a personal representative who may act on your behalf to control the privacy of your health information. Parents and guardians will generally have the right to control the privacy of health information about minors unless the minors are permitted by law to act on their own behalf.

11. **How to Learn About Special Protections for HIV, Alcohol and Substance Abuse, Mental Health and Genetic Information.** Special privacy protections apply to HIV-related information, alcohol and substance abuse treatment information, mental health information, psychotherapy notes, and genetic information.

12. **How to Obtain a Copy of Revised Notice.** We may change our privacy practices from time to time. If we do, we will revise this notice so you will have an accurate summary of our practices. You will be able to obtain your own copy of the revised notice by accessing our website or by calling your doctor's office. You may also ask for one at the time of your next visit. The effective date of the notice is noted in the top right corner of each page. We are required to abide by the terms of the notice that is currently in effect.

13. **How to Obtain a Copy of this Notice.** If you have not already received one, you have the right to a paper copy of this notice. You may request a paper copy at any time, even if you previously agreed to receive this notice electronically. You can request a copy of the privacy notice directly from your doctor's office.

14. **How to File a Complaint.** If you believe your privacy rights have been violated, you may file a complaint with us or with the Secretary of the United States Department of Health and Human Services. To file a complaint with us, please contact our Privacy Officer.

No one will retaliate or take action against you for filing a complaint.

Notice of Privacy Practices (NPP)

Covered entities must state their policies and procedures in a document called the Notice of Privacy Practices (NPP). They must also make their NPPs available on request to any person who requests them. If the CE is a health care provider with a physical service delivery site, it must have the notice available at the site for individuals to take with them.

CEs must also give each patient a Notice of Privacy Practices at the first contact or encounter. For example, health plans must comply with specific requirements for notifying enrollees in their plans.

To meet this requirement, physician practices give patients their NPPs. The notice explains how patients' PHI may be used and describes their rights. Practices may choose to use a layered approach to giving patients the notice. On top of the information packet is a short notice, like the one shown in Figure 2-2, that briefly describes the uses and disclosures of PHI and the person's rights. The longer notice is placed beneath it.

If the first service delivery to an individual is electronic, the CE must provide the electronic notice automatically in response to the individual's first request for service. For example, the first time an individual requests a refill of a prescription through a covered Internet pharmacy, the pharmacy must respond with the pharmacy's Notice of Privacy Practices. Individuals who receive electronic notices have the right to obtain paper copies on request.

Acknowledgment of Receipt-of Notice of Privacy Practices

Since providers must inform each patient about their privacy practices one time, it is important for HIPAA compliance to document this action. The most common method is to give the patient a copy of the NPP to read and then to have the patient sign a separate from called an Acknowledgment of Receipt of Notice of Privacy Practices(see Figure 2-3). This form states that the patient has read the privacy practices and understands how the provider intends to protect the patient's rights to privacy under HIPAA.

The provider must make a good-faith effort to have patients sign this document. The provider must also document-in the medical record-whether the patient signed the form. The format for the acknowledgment is up to the provider.

Example: A patient who has not received a privacy notice or signed an acknowledgment calls for a prescription refill. The office mails the patient a copy of the privacy notice, along with an acknowledgment of receipt form, and documents the mailing to show a good-faith effort that meets the office's HIPPAA obligation in the event that the patient does not return the signed form.

Only a direct provider, one who directly treats the patient, is required to have patients sign an acknowledgment. An indirect provider, such as a pathologist, must have a privacy notice but does not have to secure additional acknowledgments.

HIPAA does not require the parent or guardian of a minor to sign. If a child is accompanied by a parent or guardian who is completing other paperwork on behalf of the minor, it is reasonable to ask that adult to sign the acknowledgment of receipt. On the other hand, if the child or teen is unaccompanied, the minor patient may be asked to sign.

Thinking it Through

Answer these questions based on the information in Figure 2-2.

1. What document is required when a patient asks ABC Clinic to transfer a record to another person or organization?

2. Is written authorization from a patient needed to use or disclose health information in an emergency?

3. What is the purpose of an accounting of disclosures?

Figure 2-3: Sample Acknowledgment Receipt of Notice of Privacy Practices

I understand that the providers of ABC Clinic may share my health information for treatment, billing, and health care operations. I have been given a copy of the organization's notice of privacy practices that describes how my health information is used and shared. I understand that ABC Clinic has the right to change this notice at any time. I may obtain a current copy by contacting the practice's office or by visiting the website at www.xxx.com.

My signature below constitutes my acknowledgment that I have been provided with a copy of the notice privacy practices.

Signature of Patient or Legal Representative Date

If signed by legal representative, relationship to patient:

Disclosure of PHI

Under the HIPAA privacy standards, providers do not need specific authorization in order to use or disclose patients' PHI for treatment, payment, and operations (TPO) purposes, but they do need permission to release information for other reasons. Use of PHI means sharing or analysis within the entity that holds the information. Disclosure means the release, transfer, provision of access to, or divulging of PHI outside the entity holding the information. State law varies concerning whether just the fact of a case is to be reported or if the patient's name must also be reported. The practice guidelines reflect the state laws and must be strictly observed, as all these regulations should be, to protect patients' privacy and to comply with the regulations.

Research Data

PHI may be made available to researches approved by the CE. For example, if a physician is conducting clinical research on a type of diabetes, the practice may share information from appropriate records or analysis. When the researcher issues reports or studies based on the information, specific patients' names may not be identified.

Research subjects have the same rights as clinical care patients. That they can access the study's designated record set-most often a duplicate of the clinical record. They typically do not have the right to access the proprietary data of the study sponsor or any data that would compromise the integrity of the research.

Other Exceptions

Patients who are in the custody of correctional institutions or law enforcement personnel are another exception to the usual privacy standards for release of PHI without authorization. The covered entity can release information if law enforcement officers are investigating a crime or think that a patient is a crime victim. Likewise, PHI may be released for national security, intelligence, or other essential government purposes.

Psychotherapy Notes

Psychotherapy notes have special protection under HIPAA. According of the American Health Information Management Association Practice Brief on Legal Process and Electronic Health Records:

Under the HIPAA Privacy Rule, psychotherapy notes are those recorded (in any medium) by a healthcare provider who is a mental health professional documenting or analyzing the content of conversation during a private counseling session or a group, joint, or family counseling session and that are separated from the rest of the individual's medical record. Notes exclude medication prescription and monitoring, counseling session start or stop times, the modalities and frequencies of treatment furnished, results of clinical tests, and any summary of diagnosis, functional status, the treatment plan, symptoms, prognosis, and progress to date. The privacy rule gives such notes extra protection, as may state law. (www.ahima.org.)

Psychotherapy notes cannot contain general notes, such as prescriptions, laboratory test results, or progress notes; they are the subjective notes of the psychiatrist. Summary information covering the patient's current mental state, medications, and other information needed for treatment or payment is regularly placed in the patient's medical records.

State Statutes

Some state statues are more stringent than HIPAA specifications. Areas in which state statues may differ from HIPAA include the following:

- Designated record set

- Psychotherapy notes

- Rights of inmates

- Information complied for civil, criminal, or administrative court cases

Each practice's privacy official reviews state laws and develops policies and procedures for compliance with the HIPAA Privacy Rule. The tougher rules are implemented.

IINCIDENTAL USE AND DISCLOSURE

The privacy standards do not prohibit an incidental use and disclosure, meaning a release of PHI that happens as a result of (incident to) a correct us or disclosure.

Examples: A provider instructs an administrative staff member to bill a patient for a particular procedure and is overheard by someone in the waiting room.

A health plan employee discussing a patient's health care claim on the phone is overheard by another employee who is not authorized to handle patient information.

If the provider and the health plan employee in these examples made reasonable efforts to avoid being overheard and reasonable limited the information shared, and incidental use or disclosure resulting from their conversations would be allowed under the Privacy Rule.

Thinking It Through

Based on your knowledge of the HIPAA Privacy Rule, do you think each of the following actions is compliant?

1. A medical insurance specialist does not disclose a patient's history of cancer on a workers' compensation claim for a sprained ankle. Only the information the recipient needs to know is given.

2. A physicians' assistant faxes appropriate patient cardiology test results before scheduled surgery.

3. A physician sends an e-mail message to another physician requesting a consultation on a patient's case.

4. A hospital notifies a patients' adult child that his father has suffered a stroke and is in the intensive care unit.

Patients' Rights

Within the covered entity's designated record set, patients have the right to:

- Access, copy, and inspect their PHI

- Request amendments to their health information

- Obtain accounting of most disclosures of their health information

- Receive communications from providers via other means, such as sending a communication in a closed envelope but no on a postcard

- Complain about alleged violations of the regulations and the provider's own information policies

- Request restrictions on uses or disclosures of their PHI

ACCESS, COPY, AND INSPECT

The covered entity must permit individuals to access, copy, and read their PHI held both by the CE and by any business associates. Access should generally be provided within thirty days. This period may be extended another thirty days by providing an explanation to the patient.

The CE may charge reasonable cost-based fees for copies of records. The fee may include only the cost of copying (including supplies and labor) and postage, if the patient requests that the copy be mailed. If the patient has agreed to receive a summary or explanation of protected health information, the CE may also charge a fee for preparation of the summary or explanation. The fee may not include costs associated with searching for and retrieving the request information.

Various state laws also control the fees providers can charge a patient for copies of their medical records. Since a CE can charge only "reasonable" cost-based fees for providing medical records to patients, fees that are not cost-based, even if permitted by a state statue, may be contrary to the HIPAA regulation and thus preempted.

AMENDMENTS

An amendment is the correction of a finalized entry in a medical record that has been identified as incorrect. Corrections are in fact part of the medical record, so regular documentation guidelines must be followed when they are made. HIPAA requires covered entities to have a policy to meet HIPAA rules for accepting and processing patient's requests to amend their records. These guidelines require CEs to review and answer requests within a thirty-day period if the records are accessible on-site, or within sixty days if stored off-site. Many CEs design an amendment form for patients to use. Some requests for amendment address factual matters, such as an incorrect birthday. Others, however, are more difficult to resolve because patients differ with the terminology used by the provider, which is essentially subjective and a professional judgment of the provider. Such issues are worked out through an amendment process. The CE can deny a request for amendment if the item is accurate and complete, or if it is not part of the designated record set and would not be available for the patient's access under the Privacy Rule.

Table 2-2 AMIA/AHIMA Principles on Confidentiality of PHI

- Inform individuals, through clear communications, about their rights and obligations and the laws and regulations governing protection and PHI use.

- Notify individuals in clear language about the organization's privacy practices and their rights in cases of breaches.

- Provide individuals with a convenient, affordable mechanism to inspect, copy, or amend their identified health information/records.

- Protect PHI confidentiality to the fullest extent prescribed under HIPAA, regardless of whether the organization and its employees all comply with HIPAA, state laws, and the policies and procedures in place to protect PHI.

- Use PHI only for legitimate purposes as defined under HIPAA or applicable laws.

- Prohibit PHI use for discriminatory practices, including those related to insurance coverage or employment decisions.

- Timely notification of individuals if security breaches have compromised the confidentiality of their PHI.

- Work with appropriate law enforcement to prosecute to the maximum extent allowable by law any individual or organization who intentionally misuses PHI.

- Continuously improve processes, procedures, education, and technology so PHI practices improve over time.

Source: American Medical Informatics Association and American Health Information Management Association Position Statement, quoted in For the Record, October 16, 2006.

ACCOUNTING FOR DISCLOSURES

Patients have the right to an accounting of disclosures (see Figure 2-5) of their PHI. The list of disclosures does not have to include release:

- For TPO

- To the individual who is making the request (or to the individual's representative)

- For notification of or to persons involved in an individual's health care or payment for health care, for disaster relief, or for facility directories

- If the patient has signed an authorization to release the information

- Of a limited data set, such as for research

- For national security

- To correctional institutions or law enforcement officials

- Incident to otherwise correct release

When a patient's PHI is accidentally disclosed externally-to an outside person or organization-the disclosure should be documented in the individual's medical record, since the individual did not authorize it and it was not a permitted disclosure. An example is faxing a discharge summary to the wrong physician's office. HIPAA does not require an accounting for internal appropriate cases. However, if there is a chance that the disclosure could harm the patient, best practice is to notify the patient whose records have been released, explain what happened, and describe the steps that are being taken to handle it.

CONFIDENTIAL COMMUNICATIONS REQUIREMENTS

Patients have the right to ask covered entities to communicate with them in a way that is not the CE's usual procedure. For example, an individual may ask a provider to use particular address or phone number, perhaps preferring contact at home or at the office. Health plans, specifically, must accommodate patients who indicate that disclosing their PHI could harm them and must follow their instructions for confidential communication.

PATIENT COMPLAINTS

Patients who observe privacy problems in their providers' offices can complain to the provider or the health plan,or to the Office for Civil Rights (OCR). Complaints to OCR must be in writing and sent either on paper or electronically, as described in Figure 2-6. They must be filed within 180 days of when the complaint knew or should have known that the act had occurred. In addition, after the compliance dates above, individuals have a right to file a complaint directly with the covered entity. Individuals should refer to the covered entity's Notice of Privacy Practices for more information about how to file a complaint with the covered entity.

REQUESTS FOR RESTRICTIONS

A covered entity must permit an individual to ask the CE to restrict uses or disclosures of protected health information about the individual to carry out treatment, payment, or health care operations. A CE is not required to agree to a restriction. If the CE agrees to the restriction, it must honor this agreement unless the person needs emergency treatment that requires the disclosure.

Thinking It Through

1. Under the HIPAA privacy standards, does accounting for disclosure information include the following?

2. Release of the record for research purposes

3. Uses of the record by the nurse who is treating the patient

4. Releases authorized by the patient

5. Release of documentation to the patient's insurance company.

Figure 2-5 Patient Request for an Accounting of Disclosure

PATIENT REQUEST FOR ACCOUNTING OF DISCLOSURES

Patient Name
Patient Address
Medical Record #   **Date of Birth**
Name & address of Requestor if not patient

Please consider this a request for an accounting of all disclosures for the time frames indicated below (Maximum time frame that can be requested is six years prior to the date of the request, but not before April 14, 2003). I understand that there is a fee for this accounting and wish to proceed. I understand that the accounting will be provided to me within sixty days unless I am notified in writing that an extension of up to thirty days is necessary."

Patient or Requestor to Complete:			Practice to Complete:	
From Date(s):	To Date(s) Purpose of Disclosure	Date	Date	Fee
Request in Info				
To pt.				
Date:		Signature of Patient or Legal Rep:		
Date:		Signature of Patient or Legal Rep:		

RELEASE OF INFORMATION FOR TREATMENT, PAYMENT, AND OPERATIONS

Employees of covered entities follow a release of information (ROI) process to access PHI, prepare it for transmission, and sent it to an individual or entity that has permission under HIPAA to obtain it.

Both use and disclosure of PHI are necessary for medical care, and so are permitted for treatment, payment, and health care operations (TPO), which are defined as follows:

- **Treatment:** This primarily consists of discussion of the patient's case with other providers. For example, a physician may document the role each member of the health care team in providing care. Each team member then records actions and observations so that the ordering physician knows how the patient is responding to treatment.

- **Payment:** Providers usually submit claims to health plans on behalf of patients; this involves exchanging demographic and diagnostic information. Payment activities include determining insurance eligibility and coverage as well as billing and collections.

- **Operations:** This purpose includes activities such as accreditation (such as by the Joint Commission), staff training, and quality improvement.

Release by any Method

Information for TPO can be released by using any method of communication, including in writing, orally, by fax, or by e-mail.

PHI Release to People Acting on a Patient's Behalf

A covered entity may release PHI to a family member, a relative, a friend, or other individuals who ask for the information on the behalf of the patient. The CE must have reasonable assurance that the person has been identified by the patient as being involved in his or her care. The CE can release this information if the patient does not object. Informal permission can be obtained by asking the patient. If the patient is not present or is incapacitated, the CE can make the disclosure if it is in the best interests of the patient.

Examples: A health plan discloses relevant PHI to a beneficiary's daughter who has called to assist her hospitalized elderly mother with a payment issue.

A pharmacist dispenses filled prescriptions to a son picking up the items for his mother.

Although the HIPAA privacy standards permit sharing PHI for TPO purposes without authorization, they also require verification of the identity of the person who is asking for the information. The person's authority to access PHI must also be verified. If the requestor's right to the information is not certain, most covered entities follow a conservative policy that requires the patient to authorize the release of PHI.

People also have the right to request that they can be contacted at different places or in different ways. Patients may ask to be called at home rather that at the office, or to have written communications sent in an envelope rather than on a postcard. Patients also can opt out of facility directories; these individuals are called "no information" patients.

Case Discussion

At the beginning of the chapter, three cases were presented. They are reviewed below, with discussion about whether the actions were HIPAA-compliant.

CASE 1

A medical insurance specialist sends a patient's asthma history to the insurance company to resolve a claim that is being questioned.

Discussion: the use of the patient's medical record to handle a health care claim for payment purposes is compliant under the HIPAA privacy standards. It does not require the patient's authorization.

CASE 2

A hospital pins patients' thank you letters to a bulletin board in the main lobby.

Discussion: Unless the hospital, as the covered entity, had permission from the patients to display their letters, this use is potentially a violation of HIPAA. Best practice is to display this kind of communications from patients in a staff-only area.

CASE 3

A hospital had treated a patient for a condition and identified the patient as having a very rare blood type. Now, another patient needs a donation of this blood type for essential surgery, but none is available in the regular blood supply. The hospital staff uses its database to identify and contact the patient with the rare blood type to ask for a blood donation.

Discussion: This action is HIPAA-compliant because the information is being sought for treatment purposes.

Figure 2-6 OCR Privacy Rule Complaint Procedure

U.S. Department of Health and Human Services* Office for Civil Rights HOW TO FILE A HEALTH INFORMATION PRIVACY COMPLAINT WITH THE OFFICE FOR CIVIL RIGHTS

If you believe that a person, agency or organization covered under the HIPAA Privacy Rule ("a covered entity") violated your (or someone else's) health information privacy rights or committed another violation of the Privacy Rule, you may file a complaint with the Office for Civil Rights (OCR). OCR has authority to receive and investigate complaints against covered entities related to the Privacy Rule. A covered entity is a health plan, health care clearinghouse, and any health care provider who conducts certain health care transactions electronically. For more information about the Privacy Rule, please look at our responses to Frequently Asked Questions (FAQs) and our Privacy Guidance. (See the web link near the bottom of this page.)

Complaints to the Office for Civil Rights must: (1) be filed in writing, either on paper or electronically; (2) name the entity that is the subject of the complaint and describe the acts or omissions believed to be in violation of the applicable requirements of the Privacy Rule; and (3) be filed within 180 days of when you knew that the act or omission complained of occurred. OCR may extend the 180-day period if you can show "good cause." Any alleged violation must have occurred on or after April 14, 2003 (on or after April 14, 2004 for small health plans), for OCR to have authority to investigate.

Anyone can file written complaint in any written format. We recommend that you use

---

the OCR Health Information, Privacy Complaint Form which can be found on our web site or at an OCR Regional office. If you prefer, you may submit a written complaint in your own format. Be sure to include the following information in your written complaint:

Your name, full address, home and work telephone numbers, email address.

If you are filing a complaint on someone's behalf, also provide the name of the person on whose behalf you are filing.

Name, full address and phone of the person, agency or organization you believe violated you (or someone else's)health information privacy rights or committed another violation of the Privacy Rule.

Briefly describe what happened. How, why, and when do believe your (or someone else's) health information privacy rights were violated, or the Privacy Rule otherwise was violated?

Any other relevant information.

Please sign your name and date your letter.

The following information is optional.

Do you need special accommodations for us to communicate with you about this cannot reach you directly, is there someone else we can contact to help us reach you?

Have you filed your complaint somewhere else?

The Privacy Rule, developed under authority of the Health Insurance Portability and Accountability Act of 1996 (HIPAA), prohibits the alleged violating party from taking retaliatory action against anyone for filing a complaint with the Office for Civil Rights. You should notify OCR immediately in the event of any retaliatory action . . . . . .

If you require an answer regarding a general health information privacy question, please view our Frequently Asked Questions (FAQs). If you still need assistance, you may call OCR (toll-free) at: 1-866-627-7748. You may also send an email to OCRPrivacy@hhs.gov with suggestions regarding future FAQs.

Mission Statement:

Introduction to Health Career's Edition II, is a new style of text book with **Spanish translation** at the end of every chapter. Employers and educator's emphasis on opportunities for career achievement in a dynamic field faced with upward growth, and a high employment retention percentage.

In the U.S. hospitals are reporting double digit position rubrics for pharmacists, radiology technician, phlebotomist's, patient care technicians and technologist, while careers with similar education time length show decline in career longevity. For example shortages for housekeeping and maintenance staff, according to (AFT) Healthcare, a division of the American Federation of Teachers. Due to better health care and insurance, along with a higher life expectancy rates, suggest the increased demand for health care services as a whole across the board.

As rapidly as today's technology progresses and becomes more computer friendly, it has likewise spiked more students from a broader variety of backgrounds and assortments. Bringing a fresher knowledge in the technical field, understanding it has fulfilled more diagnosis imaging, along with numerous possible therapies, as well as a certificate required to perform daily career required duties. Beyond technical processing educators can also motivate the involvement of students and staff alike, in the development of various "safe skills". So now I am forced to ask myself "What does the future hold for Allied Health Care practitioners?" with help from your company, and myself, a well—trained, highly educated medical professional, and organized AFT organizers as well. The answer is "Endless opportunity with room for longevity and growth with a high career demand for the future medical workforce".

Reduction in Medical Errors

Teaching medical professionals the importance of knowing the job they are being tasked with. Staff and students together will gain a greater understanding of, the importance of learning medical terminologies and definitions. With a special focus on teaching with higher regard towards all medical and safety guidelines, and requirements. Education in medical accuracy should be the main focus along with completeness. Considering the retirement of the baby-boomers, and the potential increased need for medical care for the newly insured work force, the added healthcare system requirments could lead to a breakdown in the quality of patient care. Nationwide if we as educators fail to teach with up to date materials and teaching styles. Health care numbers like expenditures in the United States exceeding $2 trillion a year. In comparison, the federal budget is $3 trillion a year we see the United States needs to invest more in the medical field growth and development.

Medical system errors and medical staff mistakes are in large of which is avoidable as a whole. If we focus our efforts on the integrity of care and the proper preparation of health care professions, things such as career advancement, and lifelong learning can and will accrue. In the 21st the nurse's rules of caring for a patient hasn't changed. However on the contrary the nurse has. Things like extra skilled customer service skills and bi-lingual Allied Health workers as well as advanced technology make this statement true. They also implement that health care is evolving to meet the needs of the evolving world. The big question is why hasn't the text materials evolved?

What your support and financial backing can do?

Open doors for many students from secondary to post-secondary education which grasp the "soft shields" needed. Allow students access to learn medical Spanish for medical translation, which in return saves time in the medical field work environment through bridging a common language gap. Your support would also make finding these sources, as well as an array of other vital medical information including, but not limited to medical math lesson effortless for students. This knowledge will allow the doctors, nurse practioners, and other administrative to perform at upper level proficiency in professionalism and responsibility.

In conclusion, in the U.S, we have the wherewithal to confront the challenge that is medical education and training. Greater institutions, as well as industry certificate entities to ascertain skills for students and staff alike. Now I implore you potential supporter and ally, to recognize the need for quality and consistency in the development of greater medical education text and methods, by showing your support by backing, stepping up higher standards of education training, and certificates in the medical field. In doing this, not only will your contributions help to address the nursing shortage but it will also make cost more manageable and efficient.

As an educator, published author, pharmacy technician, and parent, I feel gives me a responsibility. To my Profession, students, and children, to share as much knowledge and experience that I have learned and can learn.

"Common core state standards"

"Throughout the text Students will be challenged with questions that push them to refer back to what they've read."

The college and career readiness anchor standards form the backbone of the **ELA/literacy standards**, will be taught with articulate wording, making learning enjoyable as well as educational. The **"Introduction to Health Careers II"** was developed in a way so students review many different learning modules, though not limited to, using crosswords, word searches and vocabulary. After completing the text the student will have gained and comprehensive knowledge of each chapter and its learning objective. Students will learn to use cognitive reasoning and evidence collecting skills that are essential for success in today's educational goals, career goals, and life.

The math will cover the standards required by all states that have embraced the common core math standards, and those who have yet made the decision to follow the design envisioned by **William Schmidt** and **Richard Houang**. "Therefore the development of the standards began with research-based on learning progression detailing what is known today as student's mathematical knowledge, skills, and understanding develop over time.

<u>*Subtraction of Fractions*</u>

Lesson 1

General Objective:

The Student will, with a minimum accuracy of 80%, as indicated on the final math evaluation test:

1. Subtract fractions from fractions.

2. Subtract fractions from whole numbers.

3. Subtract fractions and whole numbers from mixed fractions.

4. Subtract mixed fractions from other mixed fractions and whole numbers.

Multiplication of Fractions

Lesson 2

General Objective:

The Student will, with a minimum accuracy of 80%, as indicated on the final math evaluation test:

1. Multiply fractions by fractions.

2. Multiply fractions by mixed fractions.

3. Multiply mixed fractions or fractions by whole numbers.

4. Multiply mixed fractions by other mixed fractions

Division of Fractions

Lesson 3

General objective:

The Student will, with a minimum accuracy of 80%, as indicated on the final math evaluation test:

1. Divide fractions by fractions.

2. Divide fractions by mixed fractions.

3. Divide mixed fractions or fractions by whole numbers.

4. Divide mixed fractions by other mixed fractions

Introduction to Decimal Numbers

Lesson 4

General Objective:

The Student will, with a minimum accuracy of 80%, as indicated on the final math evaluation test:

1. Identify decimal positions.

2. Change decimals to fractions.

3. Change fractions to decimals.

4. Change decimals from numerical to word form.

5. Change decimals from word form to nu0merical form.

Addition Using Decimal Numbers

Lesson 5

General Objective:

The Student will, with a minimum accuracy of 80%, as indicated on the final math evaluation test:

1. Add decimals with decimals.

2. Add decimals with mixed decimals.

3. Add decimals with whole numbers.

4. Add decimals, mixed decimals and whole numbers.

Multiplication Using Decimals

Lesson 7

General Objective:

The Student will, with a minimum accuracy of 80%, as indicated on the final math evaluation test:

1. Multiply decimals with decimals.

2. Multiply decimals with whole numbers.

3. Multiply decimals with mixed decimals.

4. Multiply decimals, whole numbers and mixed decimals simultaneously.

Subtraction Using Decimals

Lesson 6

General Objective:

The Student will, with a minimum accuracy of 80%, as indicated on the final math evaluation test:

1. Subtract decimals from decimals.

2. Subtract decimals from whole numbers.

3. Subtract decimals from mixed fractions.

4. Subtract decimals, mixed decimals and whole numbers from each other.

<u>Division Using Decimals</u>

Lesson 8

General Objective:

The Student will, with a minimum accuracy of 80%, as indicated on the final math evaluation test:

1. Divide decimals by whole numbers.

2. Divide decimals by decimals.

3. Divide whole numbers by decimals.

4. Divide whole number dividends by whole number divisors when the divider is smaller than the divisor.

Decimals and Fractions

Lesson 8A

General Objectives:

The Student will, with a minimum accuracy of 80%, as indicated on the final math evaluation test:

1. Changing decimals to fractions.

2. Reduce to lowest terms.

3. Changing decimals to a common fraction.

4. Working with Denominate Numbers

Solving Word Problems Involving:

Whole numbers, fractions, decimals, denominate numbers and averages.

Lesson 9

Application with Word Problems

General Objectives:

The Student will with a minimum accuracy of at least 80% on the final math evaluation test:

1. Solve word problems, using the four basic math operations.

2. Solve word problems involving whole numbers, fractions, decimals, denominate numbers and finding averages.

3. Distinguish when to add, subtract, multiply or divide with word problems.

Operations with Percents

Lesson 11

General Objectives:

The student will with a minimum accuracy of at least 80% on the final math evaluation test:

1. Convert fractions to decimals and percents.

2. Convert decimals to fractions and percents.

3. Convert percents to fractions and decimals.

Solving Problems Involving Percents

Lesson 12

General Objectives:

The Student will with a minimum accuracy of at least 80% on the final math evaluation test:

1. Solve percent problems involving a missing part whole or percent.

2. Identify the appropriate math process needed to solve percent problems.

3. Solve word problems involving percents.

INTRODUCTION TO PERCENTS

To solve problems involving percents, it is often necessary to change fractions to decimals, fractions to percents, decimals to percents and percents to fractions or decimals.

In this lesson, you will learn how to convert:

1. Fractions to decimals and percents.

2. Percents to decimals and fractions.

3. Decimals to fractions and percents.

The chart below converts the following commonly used fractions to decimals and percents. The information on the chart should be memorized to help you quickly solve problems using these conversions. Some of the decimals will be rounded to the nearest thousandth.

FRACTIONS	DECIMALS	PERCENTS
1/2	.5	50%
1/4	.25	25%
3/4	.75	75%
1/3	.333	33.3%
2/3	.667	66.7%
1/8	.125	12.5%
1/5	.2	20%
4/5	.8	80%

[A] CHANGING PROPER OR IMPROPER FRACTIONS TO DECIMALS

1. *Divide the numerator by the denominator.*

2. *Round the quotient to the required position if necessary.*

EXAMPLES:

a. *2/12 = 12) 2 = .166 (round to the nearest 1000th)*

b. *3/4 = 4) 3 = .75*

Change to decimals. Round to the nearest hundredth.

1. *1/20* _____

2. *1/16* _____

3. *1/12* _____

4. *1/10* _____

5. *1/8* _____

6. *3/8* _____

7. *1/5* _____

8. *1/4* _____

9. *3/10* _____

10. *1/3* _____

[B] CHANGING MIXED FRACTIONS TO DECIMALS

1. *Convert the mixed fraction to an improper fraction.*

2. *Divide the numerator by the denominator.*

3. *Round the quotient to the required position if necessary.*

EXAMPLES:

a. *2 2/4 = 10/4 = 4) 10 = 2.5*

b. *3 2/12 = 38/12 = 12)38 = 3.167 (rounded to nearest 1000th)*

Change to decimals. Round to the nearest hundredth.

1. 3/38   _____

2. 14 2/5   _____

3. 6 1/2   _____

4. 8 3/5   _____

5. 4 5/8   _____

6. 6 2/3   _____

7. 7 7/10   _____

8. 3 3/4   _____

9. 5 4/5   _____

10. 6 5/6   _____

[C] CHANGING DECIMALS TO PERCENTS

To change a decimal to a percent, move the decimal point two places to the right of its original position and place a percent sign (%) after the last digit.

EXAMPLES:

a. 07225 = 7.225%

b. 14.345 = 1434.5%

c. 635 = 63.5%

d. 65 = 65% *

* A decimal point is not necessary if it follows the last digit of the number. See (d) above.

Change the following decimals to percents.

1. 0625   _____

2. .125   _____

3. 16678   _____

4. 14.5   _____

5. *77.25*   _____

6. *3.0625*   _____

7. *1.7*   _____

8. *.17*   _____

9. *.18559*   _____

10. *13.03*   _____

[D] CHANGING PROPER OR IMPROPER FRACTIONS TO PERCENTS

1. *Divide the numerator by the denominator.*

2. *Round the quotient to the required position if necessary.*

3. *Move the decimal point two places to the right.*

4. *Place a percent sign after its last digit.*

EXAMPLES:

a. *2/3 = 3) 2 = .666 = 67% (rounded to nearest whole percent)*

b. *6/5 = 5) 6 = 1.2 = 120%*

Change to percents. Round to nearest tenth.

1. *1/20*   _____

2. *1/6*   _____

3. *1/12*   _____

4. *1/10*   _____

5. *1/8*   _____

6. *3/8*   _____

7. *1/5*   _____

8. *1/4*   _____

9. *3/10*   _____

10. *1/3* _____

[E] CHANGING MIXED FRACTIONS TO PERCENTS

1. *Convert the mixed fraction to an improper fraction.*

2. *Divide the numerator by the denominator.*

3. *Round the quotient to the required position if necessary.*

4. *Move the decimal point two places to the right.*

5. *Place a percent sign after the last digit.*

EXAMPLES:

a. *3 1/4 = 13/4 = 4) 13 = 3.25 = 325%*

b. *2 4/5 = 14/5 = 5) 14 = 2.8 = 280%*

Change to percents. Round to nearest hundreth.

1. *3 3/8* _____

2. *14 2/5* _____

3. *6 1/2* _____

4. *8 3/5* _____

5. *4 5/8* _____

6. *6 2/3* _____

7. *7 7/10* _____

8. *3 3/4* _____

9. *5 4/5* _____

10. *6 5/6* _____

[F] CHANGING PERCENTS WITH FRACTIONS TO DECIMALS

1. *Change the mixed fraction to an improper fraction.*

2. *Divide the numerator by the denominator.*

3. *Round the quotient to the required position if necessary.*

4. *Remove the percent sign and move the decimal point two places to the left of its position.*

EXAMPLES:

a. *3 2/4% = 14/4% = 4) 14 = 3.5 = .35*

b. *4 3/5% = 23/5% = 5) 23 = 4.6 = .046*

Change to decimals. Round to nearest ten thousandth.

1. *4 1/3%* _____

2. *5 1/2%* _____

3. *6 1/20%* _____

4. *7 7/10%* _____

5. *16 1/4%* _____

6. *3 2/5%* _____

7. *123/5%* _____

8. *5 3/4%* _____

9. *11 4/5%* _____

10. *9 9/10%* _____

[G] CHANGING WHOLE PERCENTS TO FRACTIONS

1. *1. Remove the percent sign.*

2. *2. Place the numerator over 100.*

3. *3. Reduce if necessary.*

EXAMPLES:

a. *17% = 17/100*

b. *341% = 341/100 = 3 41/100*

Change whole percents to fractions.

1. 5% _____

2. 625% _____

3. 620% _____

4. 340% _____

5. 15% _____

6. 75% _____

7. 40% _____

8. 8956% _____

9. 85% _____

10. 1313% _____

[H] CHANGING MIXED PERCENTS TO FRACTIONS

1. Move the decimal points two places to the left.

2. Remove the percent sign.

3. Place the results over the value of the decimal position.

EXAMPLES:

a. 7.9% = .079 = 79/1000

b. .12% = .0012 = 12/10,000 = 3/2500 (reduced)

Change mixed percents to fraction.

1. 6.25% _____

2. 60.5% _____

3. 3.5% _____

4. 16.08% _____

5. 8.5% _____

6. 9234.5% _____

7. 42.25% _____

8. 33.2% _____

9. 15.15% _____

10. 34.8% _____

[I] CHANGING FRACTIONS OF A PERCENT TO FRACTIONS

1. Remove the percent sign.

2. Multiply the fraction by 1/100.

3. Reduce if necessary.

EXAMPLES:

a. *2/3% = 2/3 x 1/100 = 2/300 = 1/150*

b. *2/4% = 2/4 x 1/100 = 2/400 = 1/200*

Change fractions of a percent to fractions.

1. *1/4%* _____

2. *1/3%* _____

3. *1/2%* _____

4. *2/5%* _____

5. *3/5%* _____

6. *2/3%* _____

7. *3/6%* _____

8. *15/60%* _____

9. *3/4%* _____

10. *8/10%* _____

[J] CHANGING PERCENTS CONTAINING MIXED FRACTIONS TO FRACTIONS

1. Remove the percent sign.

2. Change the mixed fraction to an improper fraction.

3. Multiply the result by 1/100.

4. Reduce if necessary.

EXAMPLES:

a. 7 1/3% = 22/3 x 1/100 = 22/300 = 11/150

b. 5 1/4 = 21/4 x 1/100 = 21/400

Change percents containing mixed fractions to fractions.

1. 6 1/4%   _____

2. 12 1/2%   _____

3. 16 2/3%   _____

4. 3 1/4%   _____

5. 6 2/5%   _____

6. 15 15/60%   _____

7. 83 1/3%   _____

8. 87 1/8%   _____

9. 2/3%   _____

10. 8 4/5%   _____

REVIEW WORKSHEET 17

I. CHANGE TO PERCENTS

a.	.1	.5	.75	.25	.7
b.	.15	.29	.51	.10	.33 1/3
c.	.125	.875	.2555	.975	.1225
d.	2.5	.035	3.45	.009	45.0005

II. CHANGE TO FRACTIONS

a.	50%	25%	10%	40%	75%
b.	1%	5%	12 2/3%	37%	37 1/2%

III. CHANGE TO DECIMALS

a.	1%	12%	150%	225%	310%
b.	12 1/2%	37 1/2%	6 3/4%	6 1/2%	12 3/4%
c.	1/8%	1/5%	3 2/8%	.05%	11%

IV. CHANGE TO PERCENTS

a.	1/2	1/4	3/4	2/10	4/5
b.	4/20	5/25	6/4	7/4	1/8
c.	2 1/2	5 3/4	1 4/5	50/100	3/6

V. CHANGE TO DECIMALS

a.	*1/2%*	*1/4%*	*3/4%*	*2/10%*	*4/5%*
b.	*4/20%*	*5/30%*	*6/4%*	*7/4%*	*1/8%*
c.	*2 1/2%*	*5 3/4%*	*1 4/5%*	*50/100%*	*3/6%*

VI. CHANGE TO FRACTIONS

a.	*1/2%*	*1/4%*	*3/4%*	*2/10%*	*4/5%*
b.	*4/20%*	*5/30%*	*6/4%*	*7/4%*	*1/8%*
c.	*2 1/2%*	*5 3/4%*	*1 4/5%*	*50/100%*	*3/6%*

ANSWER KEY

	(A)	(B)	(C)	(D)	(E)
1.	.05	3.38	6.25%	5%	337.5
2.	.06	14.4	12.5%	16.7%	1440%
3.	.08	6.5	16.678%	8.3%	650%
4.	.1	8.6	1450%	10%	860%
5.	.13	4.63	7725%	12.5%	462.5
6.	.38	6.67	306.25%	37.5%	666.7
7.	.2	7.7	170%	20%	770%
8.	.25	3.75	17%	25%	375%
9.	.3	5.8	18.559%	30%	580%
10.	.33	6.83	1303%	33.3%	863.3

	(F)	(G)	(H)	(I)	(J)
1.	.0433	1/20	1/16	1/400	1/16
2.	.055	25/4	121/200	1/300	1/8
3.	0605	31/5	7/200	1/200	1/6
4.	.077	17/5	201/1250	1/250	13/400
5.	.1625	3/20	17/200	3/500	8/125
6.	.034	3/4	18469/200	1/150	61/400
7.	.126	2/5	169/400	1/200	5/6
8.	.0575	2239/25	83/250	1/400	697/800
9.	.118	17/20	303/2000	3/400	1/150
10.	.099	1313/100	87/250	1/125	11/125

Solving Problems Involving Percents

Lesson 18

General Objectives:

The student will with a minimum accuracy of at least 80% on the final math evaluation test:

A. Solve percent problems involving a missing part whole or percent.

B. Identify the appropriate math process needed to solve percent problems.

C. Solve word problems involving percents.

FINDING THE PART

UNKNOWN	PROCESS	FORMULA	EXAMPLE
PART	MULTIPLY	WHOLE X PERCENT	5% of 60 = ? 60 x .05 3 (solution)

In this part of the lesson, you will learn to solve math problems when the whole and percent are known, and the part is unknown.

When you are looking for the part, two terms are known:

The whole and the percent.

To find the PART, you should follow the steps below:

1. Determine that the part is missing.

2. Change the percent to a decimal.

3. Multiply the whole by the decimal equivalent of the percent.

EXAMPLES:

A. 50% of 24 =   STEP 1:   The part is missing
                    STEP 2:   50% = 5
                    STEP 3:   24 x .5 = (12) solution

B. 25% of 40 =   STEP 1:   The part is missing
                    STEP 2:   25% = .25
                    STEP 3:   40 x .25 = (10) solution

WORKSHEET ONE

1. 15% of 656   _____

2. 25% of 484   _____

3. 87 1/2% of 80   _____

4. 12 1/2% of 24   _____

5. 8 3/4% of 96   _____

6. 180% of 94   _____

7. 95% of 120   _____

8. 6 3/4% of 95   _____

9. 8% of 200   _____

10. 3/4% of 5000   _____

11. 37 1/2% of 960   _____

12. 125% of 950   _____

13. 8% of 325   _____

14. 6% of 66   _____

15. 2% of 88   _____

16. 5% of 95   _____

17. 200% of 19   _____

18. 27% of 936   _____

19. 40% of 440   _____

20. 2% of 7800   _____

21. .5% of 200   _____

22. 6.8% of 920   _____

23. .05% of 10000   _____

24. .12 1/2% of 600   _____

25. .3 3/4% of 500   _____

WORD PROBLEMS: FINDING THE PART

Many students have problems solving word problems involving percents.

On the following pages, you will find information showing you how to solve word problems involving finding the part.

Word problems involving finding the part, like numerical problems, use the process of multiplication and follow the same formula.

THE PART = THE PERCENT X THE WHOLE or P = % X THE WHOLE

Unlike numerical problems, word problems require the student to determine which percent is to be used to multiply the whole.

As stated earlier, percent means 100 or out of 100. If a problem states that 30% of a whole is removed, it would be logical to assume that 70% remains out of 100.

Because the percent we use to multiply the whole by must be equal to the part we are looking for, it is often necessary for us to determine whether we will be using the percent remaining or the percent removed.

The percent we use is determined by the question asked. If the question asks for the part remaining or paid, you must use the percent that is paid or remains out of 100.

A. Larry bought a $60.00 bike for 10% off. How much did he save?

In the problem above the percent that will be used is equal to the percent saved. He saved 10%, therefore we will use 10%.

B. Larry bought a $60.00 bike for 10% off. How much did he pay?

In this problem the percent that will be used is equal to the percent paid. If he saved 10%, he paid 90% since 100% = 10% + 90%.

FINDING THE PART

Mary had 30 apples. 10% of the apples were stolen. How many apples did she have remaining?

1. What process will we use? <u>MULTIPLICATION</u>

2. What is the whole equal to? <u>30 APPLES</u>

3. What are we looking for? <u>THE NUMBER OF APPLES THAT WERE NOT STOLEN.</u>

4. A whole is equal to what percent? <u>100%</u>

5. If 10% of the apples are gone out of 100%, what percent remains? <u>100%—10% = 90%</u>

Because the percent remaining is equal to the part remaining, we will multiply the whole by 90%.

$$30 \times 90\% = 30 \times .90 = 27 \quad \underline{27 \text{ apples remain}}$$

Mary had 30 apples. 10% of the apples were stolen. How many apples were stolen?

1. What process will we use? <u>MULTIPLICATION</u>

2. What is the whole equal to? <u>30 APPLES</u>

3. What are we looking for? <u>THE NUMBER OF APPLES THAT WERE STOLEN.</u>

4. A whole is equal to what percent? <u>100%</u>

5. What percent of the apples were stolen? <u>10%</u>

Because the percent remaining is equal to the part remaining, we will multiply the whole by 10%.

$$30 \times 10\% = 30 \times .10 = 3 \quad \underline{3 \text{ apples stolen}}$$

WORKSHEET TWO

1. Students sold tickets for a concert. Tickets for 90% of the 850 seats were sold in the first week. How many tickets remained to be sold.

2. Jerry bought a $2000.00 car for 20% off. How much did he pay?

3. 72% of 325 students were present today. How many students were absent?

4. Students sold tickets for a concert. The auditorium could seat 850 people. If 10% of the tickets were not sold, how many tickets were sold?

5. One day 52% of the students were absent. If the school's enrollment is 2200, how many students were present?

6. Carl's father said that he would help Carl buy a used motorcycle. He told Carl that he would pay 25% of the cost. How much must Carl pay if the motorcycle costs $525?

7. Jack is buying a used car for $1,500. He pays 40% down and will pay the remainder in installments. What amount does he owe in installments?

8. Susan takes home $750 each month. She decided to save 15% of each check. How much money will she have left to spend each month?

9. A refrigerator listed at $480 is marked 20% off at a sale. What is the sale price?

10. At a 25% off sale you purchase a television set originally marked at $695. What do you pay for the television?

11. Chuck Balding is a salesperson. He is paid commission of 2% of all the sales he makes. His company deducts 6.7% for Social Security and 20% for Federal Income Tax. If Chuck sells $23,586, how much will his check be?

12. How many problems did Joan have right if she received a grade of 85% in a mathematics test of 20 problems?

13. Richard received a grade of 60% in a spelling test of 25 words. How many words did he misspell?

14. The enrollment in the Western Junior High School is 850. If the attendance for a certain month was 92%, how many absences were there during the month?

15. A house worth $47,900 is insured for 80% of its value. How much would the owner receive if the house were destroyed by fire?

WORKSHEET THREE

1. If 2.3% of every 1,000 automobiles made in a single year were station wagons, how many were not station wagons?

2. A television set that regularly sells for $485.00 is on sale for 20% off. What is the sale price?

3. A certain school district has a budget of $500,000 to be used on all the necessary expenses. If 62.5% is spent on salaries, how much of the budget is spent on salaries?

4. How many problems did Joan have correct if she received a grade of 85% in a test containing 20 problems?

5. Larry played 142 games this year. He won 80% of the games. How many games did he lose?

6. Richard received a grade of 60% in a spelling test of 25 words. How many words did he misspell?

7. A certain bronze contains 59% copper. How many pounds of copper are in 300 lbs. of this certain bronze?

8. If the sales tax is 2%, what would the tax be on a purchase of $8.50?

9. Mr. Warner bought a camera at a 15% discount. If the regular price was $56.00, how much discount was he allowed?

10. The value of a car that cost $8000 decreased by 20% the first year. What was the value of the car after the first year?

11. The average number of points scored by the Ridge High basketball team decreased by 8%. They had been averaging 75 points per game. What was their new average?

12. The Rinaldi's average gas bill decreased by 4.5% when they moved. They had been spending about $23 per month for gas. How much are they now spending for gas? Round to the nearest cent.

13. The Steak House increased their menu prices by 6%. A complete dinner had been 12.50. What was the new price for the dinner?

14. The population of this town was 1750. The town grew by 8% over the previous year. What is the current population?

15. Mark weighed 120 pounds on his last birthday. His weight is 10% more this year. How much does he weigh?

FINDING THE MISSING WHOLE

UNKNOWN	PROCESS	FORMULA	METHOD	EXAMPLE
whole	division	part ÷ percent	percent) $$\frac{whole}{percent) \overline{part}}$$	3 is 5%? $$\frac{60\,whole}{0.5)\overline{3}}$$

In this lesson, you will learn how to find the **whole** when it is the unknown number.

When you are looking for the whole, two terms must be known:

The part and the percent.

You will recall that when we are looking for the part, the math process involved is multiplication. When looking for the *whole*, the math process is *division* The formula for finding the whole is as follows:

THE WHOLE = THE PART ÷ PERCENT

To find the whole, you must first determine that the whole is missing and then follow the procedure below:

1. Change the percent to decimal.

2. Divide the part known by the decimal equivalent of the percent.

    EXAMPLE 1: 24 is 50% of what number?

    STEP 1: 50% = .5

    STEP 2: .5) 24 = 48 (ANSWER 48)

    EXAMPLE 2: 15 is 10% of what number?

    STEP 1: 10% = .1

    STEP 2: .1) 15 = 150 (ANSWER 150)

WORKSHEET FOUR

Round all answers to the nearest hundredth. (NOTE: 1/3 = .3)

A.

1. 16% of what number is $48.00? _____

2. 31% of what number is 279? _____

3. 2.5% of what number is $5.65? _____

4. 42% of what number is $24.36? _____

5. 5 1/2 of what number is $23.00? _____

6. 65% of what number is 260? _____

7. 3 1/4 of what number is $65.50? _____

8. 33 1/3 of what number is 78? _____

9. 35% of what number is $65.20? _____

10. .3% of what number is $.65? _____

11. 5% of what number is 60? _____

12. 120% of what number is 67.2? _____

13. 20% of what number is 58? _____

B.

14. 17 is 33 1/3% of what number? _____

15. 30 is 25% of what number? _____

16. 45 is 250% of what number? _____

17. 9 is 1 1/2% of what number? _____

18. 90 is 4.5% of what number? _____

19. 48 is 150% of what number? _____

20. 6 is 8% of what number? _____

21. 21) 63 is 75% of what number? _____

22. 17 is .2% of what number?   _____

C.

23. Find the number that 27 is 15% of.   _____

24. Find the number that 12 is 6 1/4% of.   _____

25. Find the number that 1054 is 85% of.   _____

FINDING THE MISSING WHOLE

When solving word problems that involve finding the missing whole, we must determine that the whole is missing. Once we have determined that the whole is missing, we must then follow the procedure below.

STEP 1: Determine what percent the part represents.

STEP 2: Divide the part by the answer of step 1.

STEP 3: Round your answer to the requested place if necessary.

EXAMPLE 1: Larry bought a boat on sale at 25% off. He paid $300.00 for the boat. What was the original price of the boat?

1. What term is missing? THE WHOLE NUMBER

2. $300.00 represents what percent? THE PERCENT THAT HE PAID

3. If he saved 25%, what percent did he pay? HE PAID 75%

4. Divide the part (300) by 75%, and you will obtain the original price of the boat. .75 ÷ 300 = 400 ($400 is the original price)

EXAMPLE 2: Sara bought a car for $500.00. She saved 15% buying the car. How much was the car before the discount?

1. What term is missing? THE WHOLE NUMBER

2. $500.00 represents what percent? THE PERCENT THAT SHE PAID

3. If she saved 15%, what percent did she pay? SHE PAID 85% (100%-15% = 85%)

4. Divide the part (500) by 85%, and you will obtain the original price of the car. .85 ÷ 500 = 588.24 ($588.24 is the original price, rounded)

EXAMPLE 3: If 25% of a school's population is boys and the girls number 240, how many students are enrolled in the school?

1. What term is missing? THE WHOLE NUMBER

2. If 25% are boys, what percent are the girls? 75%

3. The 240 girls represent what percent? 75%

4. Divide the part (240) by 75%, and you will obtain the total number of students enrolled. .75 ÷ 240 = 320 (320 total students enrolled)

WORKSHEET FIVE

1. Perry saved $1.25, which was 62 1/2% of his allowance for the week. What was his weekly allowance?

2. Betsy bought a camera at a 20% reduction sale. If she paid $10.00, what was the regular price?

3. If the annual amount of depreciation is $170.00 based on a 2% rate of depreciation, what is the value of the property?

4. If 45% of the schools population are boys, and girls number 858, how many boys are enrolled?

5. If a dealer wants to make 25% profit on the selling price of a rug that cost him $60.00, what should the selling price be?

6. How much money must be invested at 4% to earn $1,000?

7. If ore contains 16% copper, how many tons of ore are needed to get one ton of copper?

8. A boy spent $2.00 which was 25% of his money. How much money did the boy have left?

9. In one day an organization raised $60.00, which was 25% of its quota. What was this organization's quota?

10. Gilbert bought a radio at 25% off and paid $24.00 for it. What was the original price of the radio?

11. Mr. Franklin bought a car for $3570.00. This was 15% off the original price. What was the original price?

12. Katie bought a dress for $8.00. This was 20% off the original price. What was the original price?

13. Molly bought a pair of shoes on sale at 33% off. She paid $12.00 for the shoes. What was the original price?

14. Mrs. Harper bought a painting for $6.00. That price was 75% of the original cost. What would it have cost without the discount?

15. By paying cash, Mr. Edwards got a 5% discount. He paid $950.00 for furniture. What would it have cost without the discount?

WORKSHEET SIX

1. On a test Myron got 20 questions correct for a score of 75%. How many questions were on the test?

2. Jack saved 32% on a new coat. The amount he saved was $54.00. What was the original price?

3. The Smiths paid $11,070 in taxes last year. That was 27% of their total earnings. What were their total earnings?

4. During a recent charity drive 114 people agreed to make a donation. This was 66% of the local residents contacted. How many people were contacted? (round to nearest whole)

5. Norman was at work 95% of the time over a 1-year period. If he worked 247 days, how many days in all could he have worked? (round to nearest whole)

6. Otto paid $189.23 in sales tax for a new motorcycle. If the tax rate was 5%, How much did the motorcycle cost?

7. On the first day of her bicycle trip, Karen rode 80 miles which was 2.5% of the distance she planned to ride. How many miles was she planning to ride?

8. A hospital has 51 patients which is 34% of its-total capacity. What is the hospital's total capacity?

9. Ramon has 45 college credit hours. This is 37.5% of the amount he needs to earn his degree. How much more does he need?

10. Pamela has $78.00, which is 60% of what she needs to buy a ring for her mother. How much more does she need?

11. This year Frank's yield of corn is 42 bushels per acre. This is 105% more than last year's yield. How many more bushels is this years yield than last year's?

12. Sandra's business expenses totaled $294,912, which was 72% of the business's net sales. What were the business's net sales?

13. Ramona rides the bus 12 miles to get to work. This is 96% of the distance from her house to her job. How many miles is it from her house to the bus stop?

14. Peter rents an apartment for $276.00 a month. This is 30% of his monthly income. How much of his income does he have left after he pays the rent?

15. Glenna is a real estate agent. She gets 5% commission on all of her sales. Last year she earned $22,500 in commission. What were her total sales?

FINDING THE PERCENT

UNKNOWN	PROCESS	FORMULA	METHOD	EXAMPLE
percent	division	part ÷ whole	$\dfrac{percent}{\text{whole}\,\overline{)\,\text{part}}}$	3 is what % of 60? $\dfrac{.05 = 5\%}{.60\,\overline{)\,3}}$

In this part of the lesson, you will learn to solve math problems when the part and the whole are known, and the percent is unknown.

When you are looking for the percent, two terms are known: The whole and the part.

EXAMPLE 1: 12 is what percent of 48?

1. What terms are known? THE PART (12) AND THEw WHOLE (48)

2. What term is missing? THE PERCENT

3. Divide the part by the whole.

4. Change the decimal to a percent. *.25 = 25%*

         48) 12

EXAMPLE 2: 10 is what percent of 25?

1. What terms are known? THE PART (10) AND THE WHOLE (25)

2. What term is missing? THE PERCENT

3. Divide the part by the whole.

4. Change the decimal to a percent. *.4 = 40%*

         25) 10

WORKSHEET SEVEN

1. 55 is _____% of 5.

2. 320 is _____% of 210.

3. 155 is _____% of 465.

4. 16 is what % of 80? _____

5. 3 is _____% of 5.

6. 25 is what % of 125? _____

7. 27 is what % of 36? _____

8. 9 is _____% of 20?

9. What % of 26 is 26? _____

10. 18 is what % of 16? _____

11. 8 is what % of 8? _____

12. What % of 50 is 65? _____

13. 1014 is _____% of 2535?

14. What % of 12.25 is 10? _____

15. .54 is _____% of 9?

16. .75 is what % of 18.75? _____

17. 2 1/4 is what % of 9? _____

18. What % of 4 2/3 is 3 1/2? _____

19. 2 is _____% of 1?

20. What % of 75 is 125? _____

21. 1/2 is what % of 3/4? _____

22. 9.6 is what % of 6.4? _____

23. What % of 36 is 48? _____

24. 45 is _____% of 54?

25. 85 is what % of 75? _____

REVIEW WORKSHEET 4

Round answers to the nearest hundredth or hundredth of a percent.

1. Mike bought a television set for $180, reduced from $240. What percent off the original price did he save?

2. Taxes are often discounted if paid at an early date. Jack Elan received a 3% discount on his tax bill of $180. How much tax did he pay?

3. Strawberries shrink when cooked. If they shrink 15%, how much would remain if you started with 16 pounds?

4. The sales tax in California is 6%. If you paid $5.34 in sales tax for a new suit, how much was the suit before taxes?

5. There are 13 hummingbirds, 40 parrots, and 16 tuscons in a certain bird collection. What percent of this collection do the tuscons represent?

6. Joe threw a ball 240 ft. Bob threw the ball 60% farther than Joe. How far did Bob throw the ball?

7. 3000 students are in the yard today. This represents 150% of the schools population. What is the schools regular population?

8. 30 children from the playclub attended the concert. 75% of the club members did not attend. How many members are in the club?

9. Lou sold $6.40 worth of clothing. If he received $72.00 for his sales, what percent of commission does he earn?

10. Last month our gas and light bill was $48. This month shows a decrease of 12-1/2%. How much is this months bill?

11. Larry sold $480 worth of clothing. If he received $72.00 for his sales, what was his rate of commission?

12. Mr. Graham saves $150 each month. If his annual income is $18,000, what percent of his income does he save annually?

13. Joe spends $185 a month for rent. His rent is 25% of his income. What is his income for a month?

14. Lou buys cans of soup for .20 each and sells them for .23 each. By what percent does he mark up the price?

15. There were to be 300 children on a field trip. If 20% of the children did not go, how many children attended the field trip?

16. One day 300 pupils were in school. This was 60% of all the pupils, how many pupils are there in the entire school?

17. Dan bought a $30 radio for $24. What % discount did he receive?

18. In 1988 Kim made $14,600 a year. In 1989 she got a 9% raise. How much did she make in 1989?

19. Wilbur took a spelling test and spelled 15 out of 120 words incorrectly. What percent did he get right?

20. A year ago May paid $1.35 for a gallon of milk. This year she pays 18% more than last year. How much does May pay for a gallon of milk this year?

REVIEW WORKSHEET 5

Round answers to the nearest hundredth of a percent.

1. Joe spends $185 a month for rent. His rent is 25% of his income. What is his income for the month?

2. 80% of the members of a union voted to strike. 216 members voted to strike. How many members are there in the union?

3. The sales tax in California is 6%. If you paid %5.34 in sales tax for a new suit, how much was the suit?

4. Sue gets 5% of the value of the shoes she sells. She made 97.15 in commissions. What was the value of the shoes she sold?

5. Jack weighs 150 pounds today. This is 75% of what he weighed 3 years ago. How much did he weigh 3 years ago?

6. Wilbur took a spelling test and spelled 15 out of 120 words incorrectly. What percent did he get right?

7. There are thirteen canaries, 40 parrots and 16 tucson's In a bird collection. What percent of the birds does the tucson's represent?

8. A dealer reduced the price of a new car by $1760. If the sticker price was $8,800, what percent doe the reduction represent?

9. Lou buys a can of soup for .20 each and sells them for .23 each. By what percent does he mark up the price?

10. Hal invested $450 in the stock market. After a year, his investment was worth $506.25. What percent of his original amount does his stock's present value represent?

11. In 1988 Kim made $14,600 a year. In 1989 she got a 9% raise. How much did she make in 1989?

12. A year ago May paid $1.35 for a gallon of milk. This year she paid 18% more than last year. How much does May pay for a gallon of mile this year?

13. Kim bought a $35.90 sweater at a 8% discount. How much did she save?

14. Joe threw a ball 240 ft. Bob threw the ball 60% farther than Joe. How far did Bob throw the ball?

15. John bought a sweater for $19.00. The sales tax is 6%. What was the cost of the sweater after taxes?

16. 3000 students are in the yard today. This represents 150% of the school population. What is the schools regular population?

17. Mike bought a television set for $180, reduced from $240. What percent off the original price did he save?

18. There were to be 300 children on a field trip. If 20% of the children did not go, how many children attended the field trip?

19. Six out of 36 cars are found to be defective. What percent of the cars are not defective?

20. 30 children from the playclub attended a concert. 75% of the club members did not attend. How many members are in the club?

REVIEW WORKSHEET 6

Round answers to the nearest hundredth of a percent.

1. Carol was told that she would have to pay $684 interest on a $6,300 loan. What interest rate would she have to pay?

2. Sears is offering 20% off of their $260 refrigerator. How much can you save by buying the refrigerator on sale?

3. Lois took a test with 80 questions. She answered 90% of the questions correctly. How many questions did she get wrong?

4. Sue bought a clock radio for $24.49. The sales tax is 8%. How much did she pay for the clock radio after taxes?

5. A year ago June paid .45 for a quart of milk. This year she pays 18% more than last year. How much does June pay for a quart of milk this year?

6. John bought a $5,365.00 car at 5% discount. How much did she save?

7. Reggie had 34 hits after 136 times at bat. What percent of the time did he get a hit?

8. Carol weighed 175 lbs. last year. She now weighs 119 ;lbs. What percent of her weight lose?

9. Gas at Hall's is .98 per gallon. At Joe's it costs $1.47 per gallon. What percent higher is Joe's gas?

10. Otto paid $189.23 in taxes for a motorcycle. The tax rate is 5%. How much did it cost?

11. Pam has $78, which is 60% of what she needs. How much more does she need?

12. In 1988 Kim made $14,600 a year. In 1989 she got a 9% raise. How much did she make in 1989?

13. Bill & Kim bought a house for #\$32,000. They made a down payment of 15%. Find the amount they owed after the down payment.

14. 3000 students are enrolled in school. If 30% of the students are girls, how many boys are in the school?

15. 3000 students are in the yard today. This represents 150% of the schools regular population. What is the schools regular population?

16. Wilbur took a spelling test and spelled 15 out of 120 words incorrectly. What percent did he get right?

17. There are thirteen canaries, 40 parrots and 16 tuscons in a bird collection. What percent of the bird's does the tuscons represent.

18. Hal invested $450 in the stock market. After a year, his investment was worth $506.25. What percent of his original amount does his stock's present value represent?

19. A television set was reduced by $32.48. If this represents a reduction of 70%, find the original price of the television.

20. John delivered 70% of the number of magazines he had. If he delivered 63 magazines, how many did he have left to sell?

FORWARD

INTRODUCTION TO HEALTH CARE CAREERS

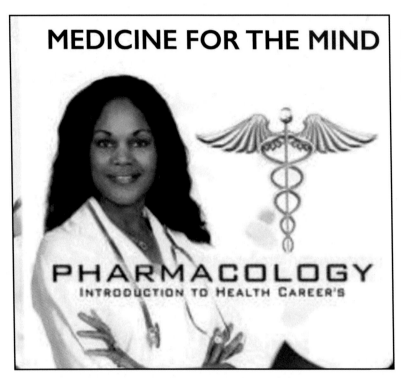

Since the earliest days of mankind, the health care provider has been one of the most respected individuals in a community. The health care provider has always been a dedicated and caring person whose number one objective has been to provide the best medical care available to their patients. Medicine has come a long way since ancient times; however, its practitioners still have one goal in common, the preservation of life. From the witch doctor, to Hippocrates, to today's doctors the health and well-being of each patient is what all health care workers strive to maintain as part of a health care team.

As modern medicine improve and expands, so does health care careers. The first doctors worked by themselves, often using family members of the sick patient to perform some of the menial duties, such as: boiling water, cleaning an area, making bandages, etc. However, as medicine became more complicated the doctors found the need to have nurses who were trained in patient care, disinfection and asepsis. The more technical medicine becomes the more health careers come into being. Improvement in laboratory techniques brought on the advent of the phlebotomist. Large hospitals, medical insurance companies and HMO's brought about the need for billing and insurance clerks.

The quest for new and better medicine made it impossible for pharmacist to fill all of their prescriptions, therefore requiring them to hire assistants, more commonly referred to as pharmacy technicians. The discovery of ether as an anesthetic made way for the anesthesiologist. In fact, the more we learn about medicine and health care the more employment opportunities open in health care.

Today, employment in the health care service field is one of the fastest growing segments in America's job market. The need for non-professional personnel is at its greatest levels in history. There is a great demand for nurses, medical receptionist, front and back office workers, billing clerks, x-ray technicians, dental assistants, pharmacy technicians, phlebotomist, laboratory assistants, sanitary engineers, and various other health care professions.

Because of the expanding health-care needs of a growing population with increasing numbers of elderly people, employment in medical-care services will greatly increase in the year to come. The Bureau of Labor Statistics has revised its labor-force projections for the 1990's. Listed among the fastest growing occupations are a number of health-related careers. Actually, the health industry is one of the largest in the United States.

Some jobs today did not exist a few years ago. For example, many jobs have resulted from the discovery of the x-ray. Today, there are even more advanced uses for x-rays. Computerized tomographic scanners are providing new jobs.

These scanners are x-ray machines that can take pictures of a section of the inside of the body without shadows from other sections interfering. Since computers are being used to study and interpret information from laboratories, people who know about them are also needed in the health field.

How should you prepare for a health career? There is no single answer to this question because there are so many different careers. Since there is a wide choice of careers the length of time needed and the place of preparation vary. For instance, other jobs have a training period that begins after high school and lasts for several weeks or months. Still others require several years of professional training. Being a physician requires a college degree in addition to years of specialized training.

The health careers that require the least amount of formal education are called entry-level careers. Some entry level health careers are those of surgical technician, EEG technologist, EKG technologist, respiratory therapy technician, clinical laboratory assistant, dietetic technician, and medical assistant.

Intermediate-level careers in health require an associate degree which can be earned in two years. Some of the intermediate-level health careers are cytotechnologist, dental hygienist, pediatric assistant, radiation-therapy technologist, licensed practical nurse, and physical-therapy assistant.

Professional-level careers in health usually require a four-year college degree, although several of these professions require additional years of education, training, and experience. Some higher-level health careers include medical technologist, speech pathologist, health educator, veterinarian, occupational therapist, registered nurse, physical therapist, and physician.

This course is designed to provide you with information to help guide you towards one of the many health care service jobs in demand and to gear you towards being an effective, efficient and knowledgeable member of a health care team.

Mrs. Edmond

GRATITUDE

This is a few words of appreciation, love, trust, and dedication to my students, friends, acquaintances and family. I have worked numerous days, months and years, to create a text book and workbook, I hope will be a learning tool a labor of love for all.

Health Careers Academy High School Stockton, Ca.

Students you gave me ideas, direction and focus to develop a product that I hope will be used to encourage all students to learn and apply gain knowledge toward a life in the health care field.

Friends and acquaintances thank you, for allowing me to talk your ears off about ideas for creating a complete text book for the health care field, with the Common Core focus. A special thanks go out to Traci Miller HCA principal, Dr. Jas Holmes, Dr. Steven West, Dr. Adam Kaye, Charline Adams, Andre Johnson(Dre), and Solominya Ivey, for your support and friendship and Many others.

To a very true friend George Law, Thank you for being you. Your always there when I need you most, truly you define friendship.

Thank you, Mom and Dad, for always believing in me. Trusting my decisions and supporting my ideas. To all of my brothers and sisters, only you know some of the challenges I faced along the way, thank you.

A very special thanks to my grandmother who will always be in my heart and be with me spiritually Mrs. Irene Jackson, your love, teaching, and guidance has carried me through life.

Printed in the United States
By Bookmasters